AF541178

Skeleton of Ox

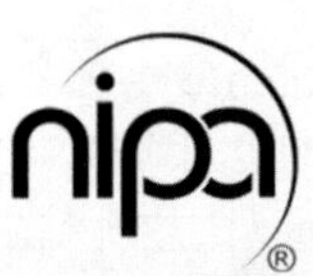

NIPA® GENX ELECTRONIC RESOURCES & SOLUTIONS P. LTD.
New Delhi-110 034

About the Author

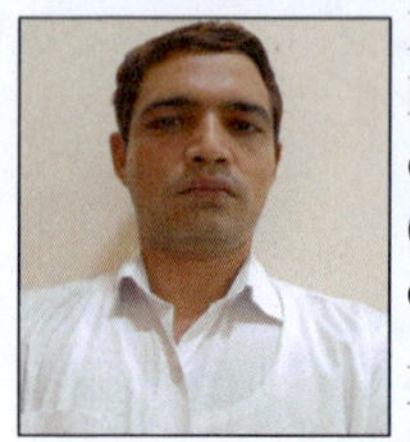

Dr. Satish Kumar Pathak is currently serving as an Assistant Professor in the Department of Veterinary Anatomy, Faculty of Veterinary and Animal Sciences, Banaras Hindu University (BHU), India. He holds over 10 years of teaching and research experience in the field of Veterinary Anatomy.

Dr. Pathak began his academic career as a Teaching Associate at the College of Veterinary and Animal Sciences, Bikaner, and later served as Assistant Professor (Contract) at the Indian Veterinary Research Institute (IVRI). Throughout his career, he has contributed significantly to veterinary anatomical sciences through both teaching and research.

He has authored 28 research papers published in reputed national and international journals. In addition to research, Dr. Pathak has contributed to academic literature as the author of one book and three book chapters.

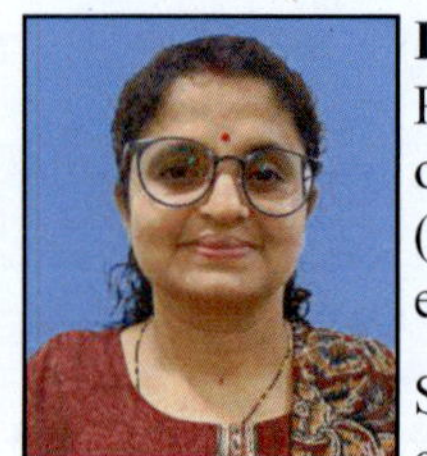

Dr. Archana Mahapatra is currently serving as an Assistant Professor in the Department of Veterinary Anatomy, Faculty of Veterinary and Animal Sciences, Banaras Hindu University (BHU). She holds over 9 years of teaching and research experience in the field of Veterinary Anatomy.

She began her academic career as an Assistant Professor (on contract) at the Department of Veterinary Anatomy, Indian Veterinary Research Institute, Bareilly, U.P. and later continued her academic tenure at BHU. Throughout her career, she has contributed significantly to veterinary anatomical sciences through both teaching and research.

She has authored 10 research papers published in reputed national and international journals. In addition to research, she has contributed to academic literature as the author of 1 book and 3 book chapters.

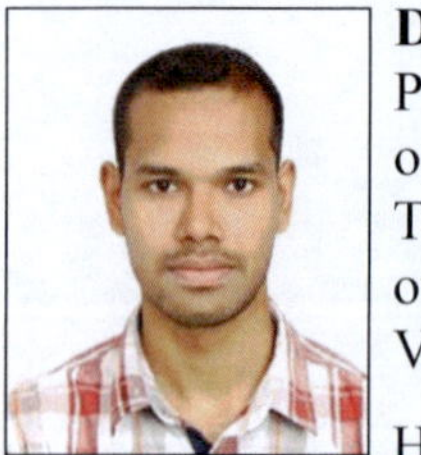

Dr. Ersavadla Rajaraviteja is currently serving as an Assistant Professor in the Department of Veterinary Anatomy, College of Veterinary Science, Mamnoor, Warangal, P. V. Narsimharao Telangana Veterinary University, Telangana, India. He holds over 8 years of teaching and research experience in the field of Veterinary Anatomy.

He began his academic career as a teaching faculty at the College of Veterinary Science, Rajendranagar, PVNRTVU, Hyderabad, Telangana, later served as an Assistant Professor at Faculty of Veterinary and Animal Sciences, Banaras Hindu University (BHU), India.

He has authored 13 research papers published in reputed national and international journals. In addition to research, he has contributed to academic literature as the author of 3 book chapters.

Skeleton of Ox
With Clinical Insights
A Colour Atlas

Satish Kumar Pathak
Assistant Professor
Department of Veterinary Anatomy
Faculty of Veterinary and Animal Sciences
Banaras Hindu University (BHU), India

Archana Mahapatra
Assistant Professor
Department of Veterinary Anatomy
Faculty of Veterinary and Animal Sciences
Banaras Hindu University (BHU), India

E. Rajaraviteja
Assistant Professor
Department of Veterinary Anatomy
College of Veterinary Science, Mamnoor, Warangal
P. V. Narsimharao Telangana Veterinary University
Telangana, India

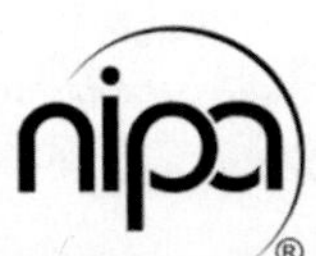

NIPA® GENX ELECTRONIC RESOURCES & SOLUTIONS P. LTD.
New Delhi-110 034

NIPA® GENX ELECTRONIC
RESOURCES & SOLUTIONS P. LTD.
101,103, Vikas Surya Plaza, CU Block
L.S.C.Market, Pitam Pura, New Delhi-110 034
Ph : +91 11 4386 0225, 9717133558, 9540816132
E-mail: newindiapublishingagency@gmail.com
Website: www.niparesources.com

Print ISBN: 978-93-58871-42-5

ebook ISBN: 978-93-58871-63-0

Composed and Designed by NIPA®.

Preface

With great enthusiasm, we present the second edition of Skeleton of Ox: With Clinical Insights: A Colour Atlas. This revised version builds upon the solid foundation of the first edition, integrating valuable feedback and thoughtful updates to further enrich its relevance and practical utility.

Our primary objective remains steadfast: to provide a comprehensive visual and anatomical guide to the intricate skeletal structure of the ox. By combining high-quality, meticulously captured photographs from multiple angles with concise textual descriptions, this atlas aims to offer a holistic and accessible understanding of bovine osteology.

The motivation to produce a second edition stemmed from our continued commitment to meet the evolving needs of undergraduate and postgraduate veterinary students, as well as researchers and educators in the field of animal anatomy. We are grateful for the encouraging response and support the first edition received, which has inspired us to refine and expand the content for this new edition.

In this edition, we have made a conscious effort to address gaps identified in the earlier version, while preserving the clarity and visual strength that characterized the original work. That said, we humbly acknowledge that no book is ever truly complete, and we welcome constructive feedback to further enhance future iterations.

We are especially thankful to New India Publishing Agency for their support in bringing this second edition to fruition, marking a significant step forward from our self-published first edition. Their professional guidance and collaboration have been instrumental in elevating the quality and reach of this work.

Finally, we extend our sincere gratitude to all those who contributed to the development of this atlas. We hope that this edition will continue to serve as a valuable resource, facilitating a deeper and more clinically relevant understanding of ox anatomy for years to come.

Authors

Contents

Appendicular Skeleton

The cattle skeleton, like that of other mammals, is a complex structure that provides support, protection, and mobility. The skeleton for study purposes is divided into two main parts: the axial skeleton and the appendicular skeleton. The axial skeleton forms the central axis of the body and includes bones such as the skull, vertebral column, ribs, and sternum. The appendicular skeleton comprises the bones of the forelimb (scapula, humerus, radius-ulna, carpals, metacarpals and phalanges) and hindlimb (os coxae, femur, patella, tibia-fibula, tarsals, metatarsals and phalanges).

Bones of Fore Limb

Key Features

- Adaptations for Grazing: The skeleton is designed for stability and endurance, with strong limb bones to support the animal's weight and a flexible neck for grazing.
- Hooves: Cattle are even-toed ungulates (order Artiodactyla), with weight distributed across two functional toes (III and IV) per hoof, supported by robust phalanges and sesamoid bones for shock absorption.
- Joints: Synovial joints (e.g., shoulder, hip, and stifle) allow mobility, while ligaments and cartilage provide stability, critical for locomotion on varied terrain.

Scapula

- **Two Surfaces**

  a) Lateral

  b) Medial

- **Three Borders**

  a) Cranial

  b) Caudal

  c) Vertebral

- **Three Angles**

  a) Cervical

  b) Dorsal

  c) Glenoid

- **Lateral Surface**

  a) Spine

  b) Supraspinous Fossa

  c) Infraspinous Fossa

  d) Acromion Process

Medial Surface

  a) Subscapular Fossa

  b) Area for the attachment of Serratus Cervicis

  c) Area for the attachment of Serratus Thoracic

- **Distal Extremity**

  a) Glenoid Cavity

  b) Tuber Scapulae

  c) Coracoid Process

  d) Glenoid Notch

Scapula (Lateral Surface)

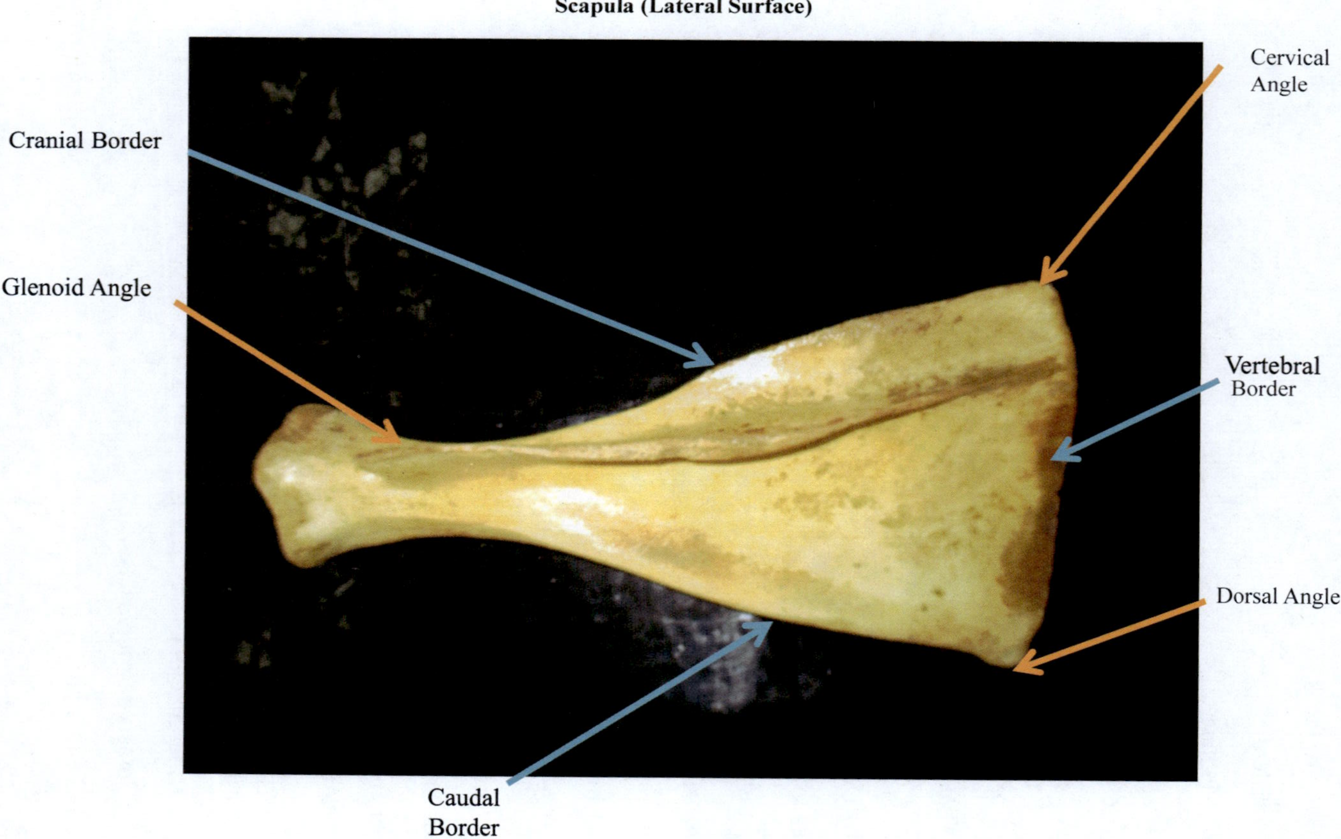

Lateral aspect of the scapula

The supraspinous fossa of the scapula houses the supraspinatus muscle, while the infraspinous fossa accommodates the infraspinatus muscle. The scapular spine serves as a prominent landmark, separating these two fossae. The scapular spine provides origin point for part of the deltoid muscle and insertion points for extrinsic shoulder muscles like trapezius and omotransversarius. The caudal border provides attachment points for both the deltoid muscle and the long head of the triceps muscle. The dorsal border is associated with the scapular cartilage. The tuber scapulae, visible from the glenoid angle on the lateral surface and positioned cranially to the glenoid cavity, serves as the origin point for the biceps brachii muscle. Teres minor muscle originated from the infraspinous fossa distally close to the caudal border.

Clinically salient features

- Scapular spine was the palpable bony prominence in the region of the shoulder girdle.
- Suprascapular nerve injury commonly referred to as "Sweeny," results in a prominent scapular spine due to atrophy of the supraspinatus and infraspinatus muscles.
- Cranial border of the scapula provides axis for the palpation of prescapular lymph node.
- Caudal angle and caudal border of the scapula form the base of the caudal lung field
- Suprascapular nerve block site: Insert the needle just above the cranial border of the scapula at the junction of the scapular spine and the cranial border. This site allows access to the suprascapular nerve as it curves around the cranial edge of the scapula.

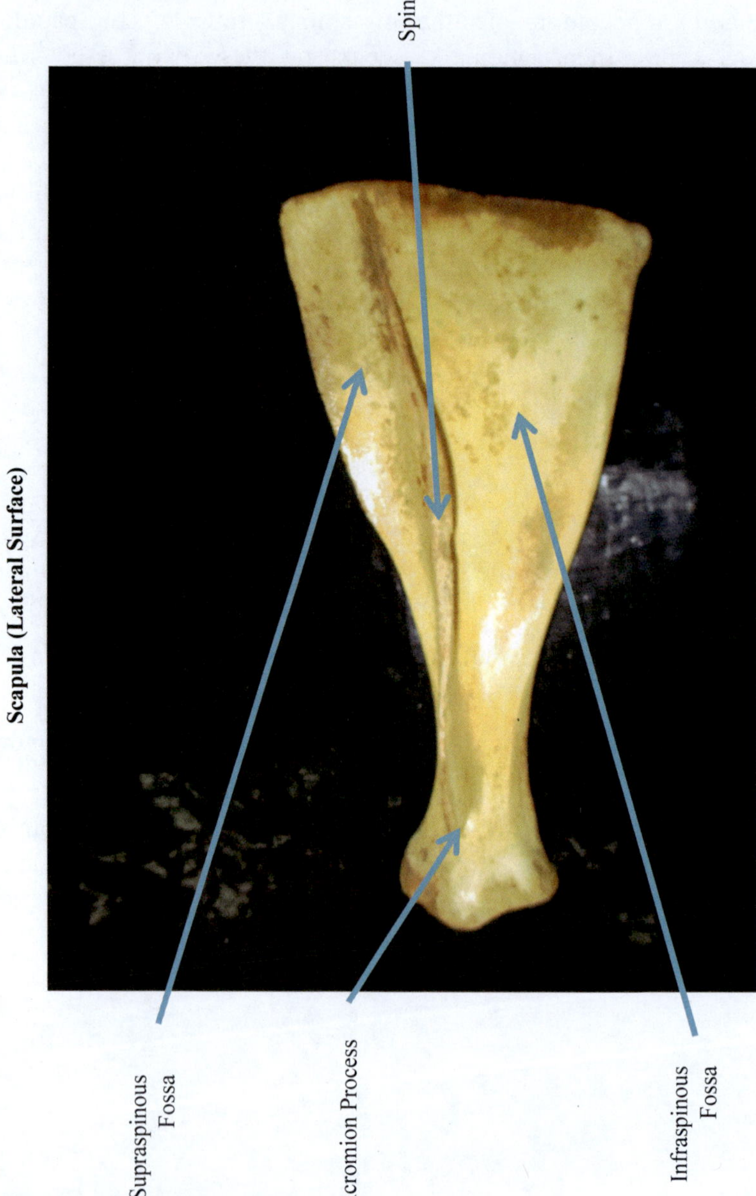

Scapula (Lateral Surface)

Fracture prone sites in the lateral aspect of scapula

Scapular Body Fractures: These fractures can be either transverse (horizontal break) or oblique (angled break). They may be non-displaced (bone pieces remain aligned) or displaced (bone fragments move out of position).

Scapular Spine Fractures: Easily palpable due to its superficial position. It affects muscle attachments and impairs the movement in the shoulder region.

Acromion Process Fractures: Tip of the Acromion process is more prone for fracture. It affects the movement created by the muscle deltoideus.

Nerve block in the lateral aspect of scapula

Suprascapular Nerve Block

Key Landmarks: Spine of the scapula and cranial border of the scapula

Site of needle insertion

- The insertion site is typically located about one-third of the way down from the top (dorsal) part of the scapula, just above the cranial border of the scapula, approximately at the point where the scapular spine and cranial border meet.
- Angle the needle slightly medially and direct it toward the neck of the scapula, where the suprascapular nerve is positioned.

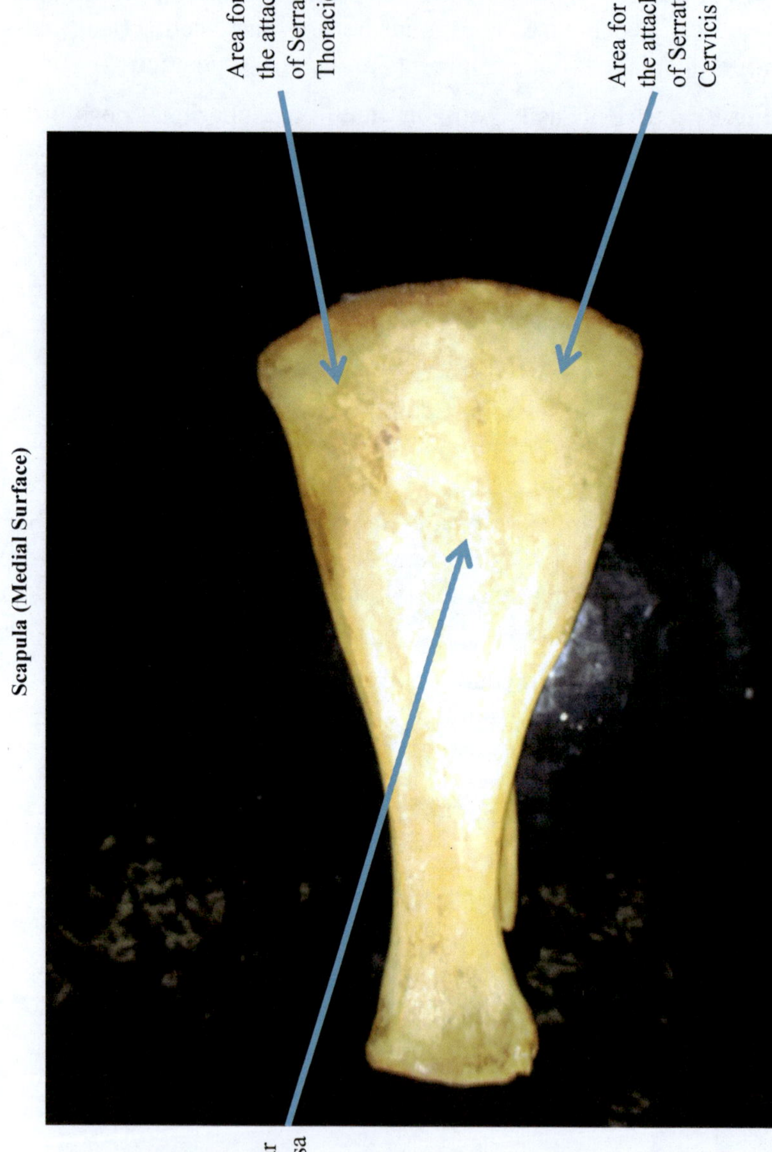

Scapula (Medial Surface)

Medial aspect of the scapula

The medial surface of the scapula, specifically the subscapular fossa is shallow and provides attachment for the subscapularis muscle, while the rough area is the site for the teres major muscle. Triangular rough areas of medial surface provide insertion point for the extrinsic shoulder muscle serratus ventralis (the cranial part is cervicis and the caudal part is thoracic). Serratus ventralis muscle keeps the scapula close to the thorax and gives stability to the scapula during the locomaotion.

Fracture prone sites in the medial aspect of scapula

Scapular Body Fractures: These fractures can be either transverse (horizontal break) or oblique (angled break). They may be non-displaced (bone pieces remain aligned) or displaced (bone fragments move out of position).

Nerve block in the medial aspect of scapula

Subscapular Nerve Block

Key Landmarks: scapular spine, cranial border of the scapula, C6 – C7 vertebrae and axilla or armpit region.

Site of needle insertion

- Insert the needle medial to the shoulder joint, in the axillary region approximately below and medial to the shoulder joint.
- The needle should be directed to reach the subscapular fossa.

Scapula (Distal Extremity)

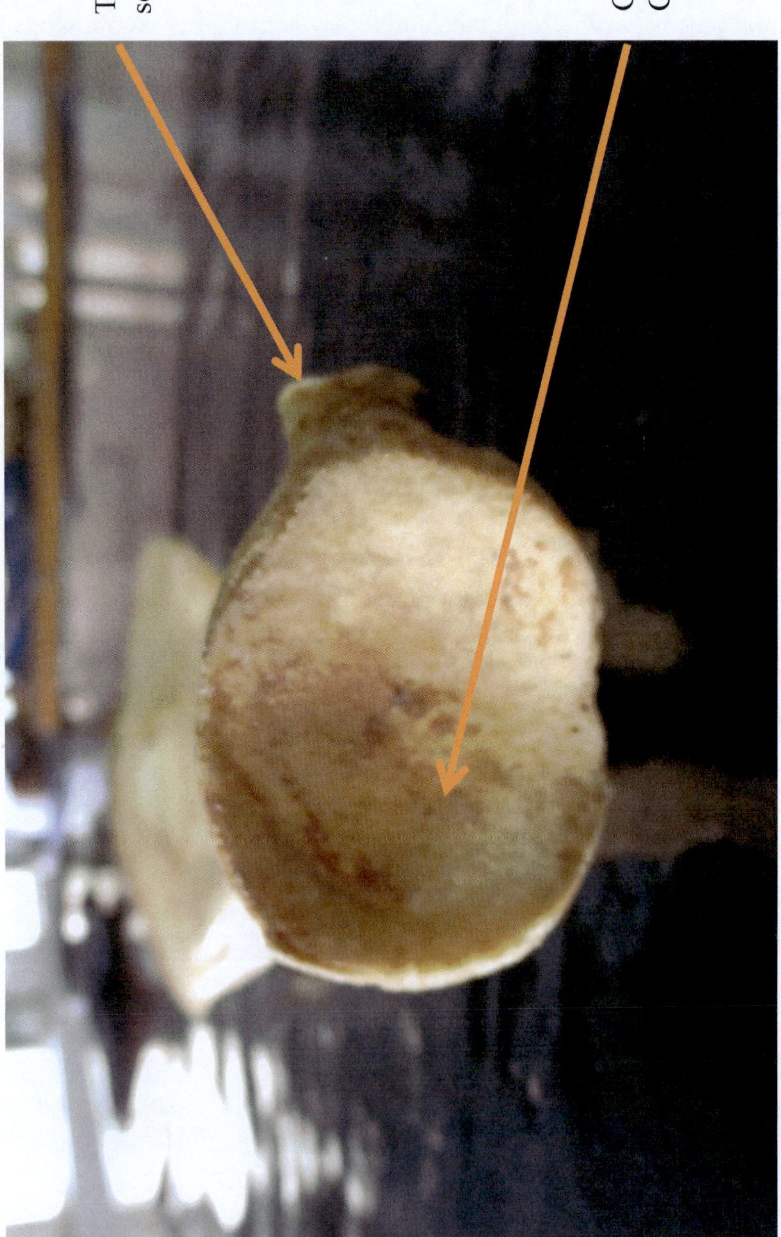

Distal Extremity of the Scapula

The distal extremity of the scapula features a shallow, cup-like depression known as the glenoid cavity and a bony prominence termed the tuber scapulae or supraglenoid tubercle. The glenoid cavity serves as the articular surface, where it forms the shoulder joint by articulating with the head of the humerus, allowing for a wide range of motion in the forelimb.

Tuber scapulae are positioned superiocranially to the glenoid cavity. A significant portion of the tuber scapulae serves as the origin point for the biceps brachii muscle. Medially, it features a small, beak-like bony projection known as the coracoid process. The coracoid process provides the origin point for the coracobrachialis muscle, contributing to shoulder joint stability and movement.

Scapula (Distal Extremity)

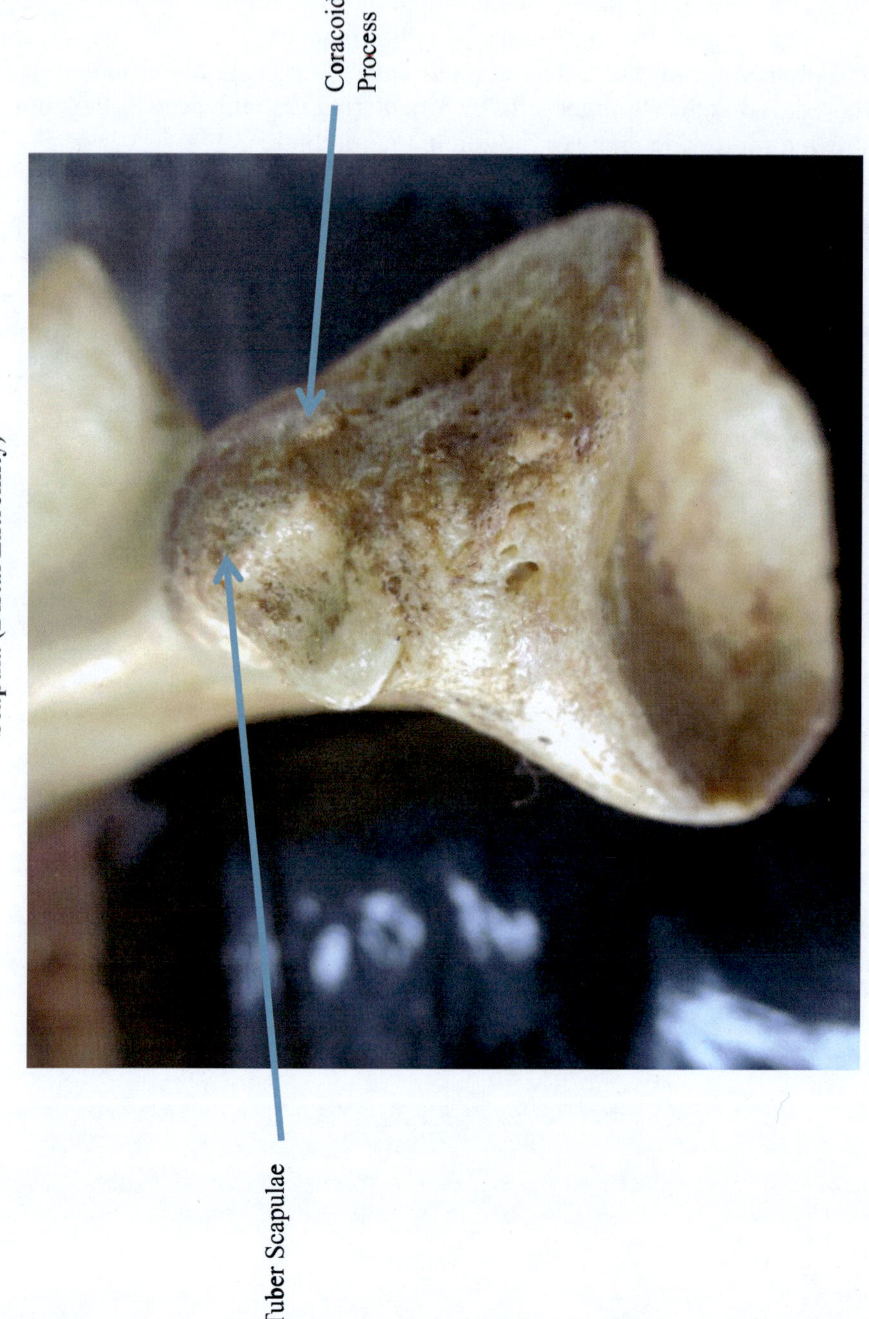

Fracture prone sites in the distal extremity of the scapula

Scapular Neck Fractures: It compromises the stability of shoulder joint.

Supraglenoid Tubercle Fractures: These fractures can impair the function of the muscle biceps brachii, leading to reduced forelimb mobility.

Glenoid Fractures: These fractures often disrupt the shoulder joint and may be associated with shoulder luxation (dislocation).

The Different Types of Scapular Fractures in Cattle

1. **Scapular Body Fractures:** These fractures can be either transverse (horizontal break) or oblique (angled break). They may be non-displaced (bone pieces remain aligned) or displaced (bone fragments move out of position).
2. **Scapular Spine Fractures:** Easily palpable due to its superficial position. It affects muscle attachments and impairs the movement in the shoulder region.
3. **Acromion Process Fractures:** Tip of the Acromion process is more prone for fracture. It affects the movement created by the muscle deltoideus.
4. **Scapular Neck Fractures:** It compromises the stability of shoulder joint
5. **Supraglenoid Tubercle Fractures:** These fractures can impair the function of the muscle biceps brachii, leading to reduced forelimb
6. **Glenoid Fractures:** These fractures often disrupt the shoulder joint and may be associated with shoulder luxation (dislocation).

- White muscle disease (nutritional myopathy due to selenium/vitamin E deficiency) can cause degeneration in muscles surrounding the scapula
- In postmortem exams, it's a key area to assess for muscle lesions, bruising, or injection damage that may affect carcass grading.
- In young calves, especially under poor hygiene conditions, hematogenous osteomyelitis may localize to bones like the scapula. It can result in localized swelling, pain, fever, and systemic illness.
- The spine of the scapula is a key anatomical landmark during clinical exams: used to assess body condition (especially muscle mass), assists in localizing shoulder lameness and useful for nerve blocks or identifying abnormal swellings mobility.

Humerus

• Proximal Extremity

a) Head

b) Neck

c) Lateral Tuberosity (two parts- summit and convexity)

d) Medial Tuberosity (two parts- cranial and caudal)

e) Bicipital Groove

f) Rough area for the tendon of Infraspinatus muscle (on lateral tuberosity)

• Distal Extremity

a) Coronoid Fossa (Cranial)

b) Olecranon Fossa (Caudal)

c) Lateral and Medial Condyles

d) Lateral and Medial Epicondyles

e) Sagittal Ridge

Humerus (Cranial Surface)

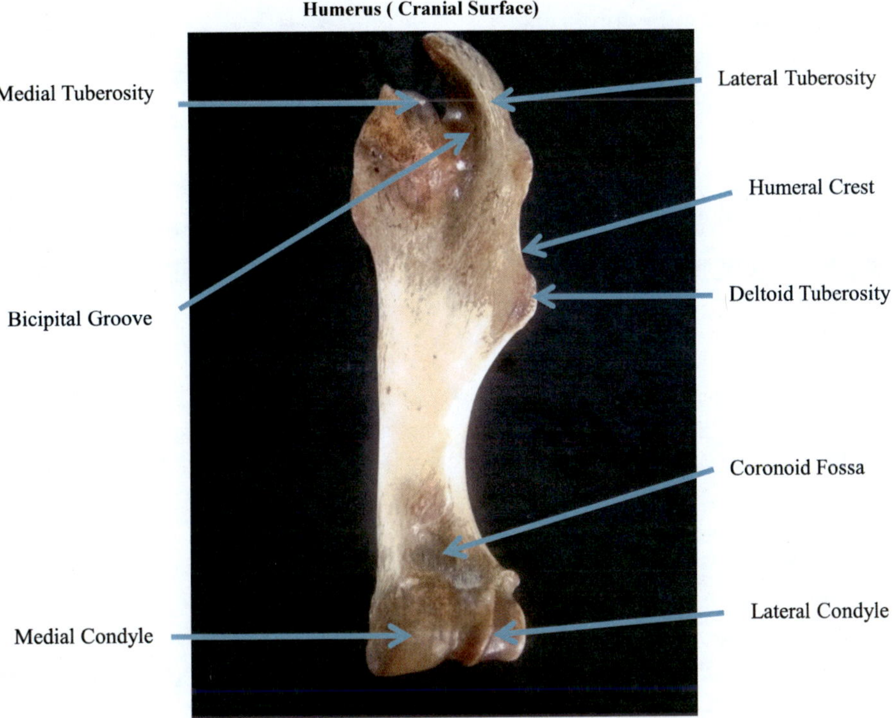

Humerus - Proximal End

At the proximal end, the cranial surface of the humerus features two prominent bony structures:

- The greater tubercle is located laterally and extends cranially, providing attachment for the supraspinatus and infraspinatus muscles. These muscles are involved in stabilizing the shoulder joint and assisting in the extension of the forelimb.
- The lesser tubercle is situated medially, offering an attachment point for the subscapularis muscle, which plays a critical role in shoulder adduction and medial rotation.

Between these tubercles lies the intertubercular (bicipital) groove, through which the tendon of the biceps brachii muscle passes. The bicipital bursa located underneath the tendon of the biceps brachii in the bicipital groove. The bicipital groove can be used as a landmark on ultrasound.

Humerus (Caudo-medial View)

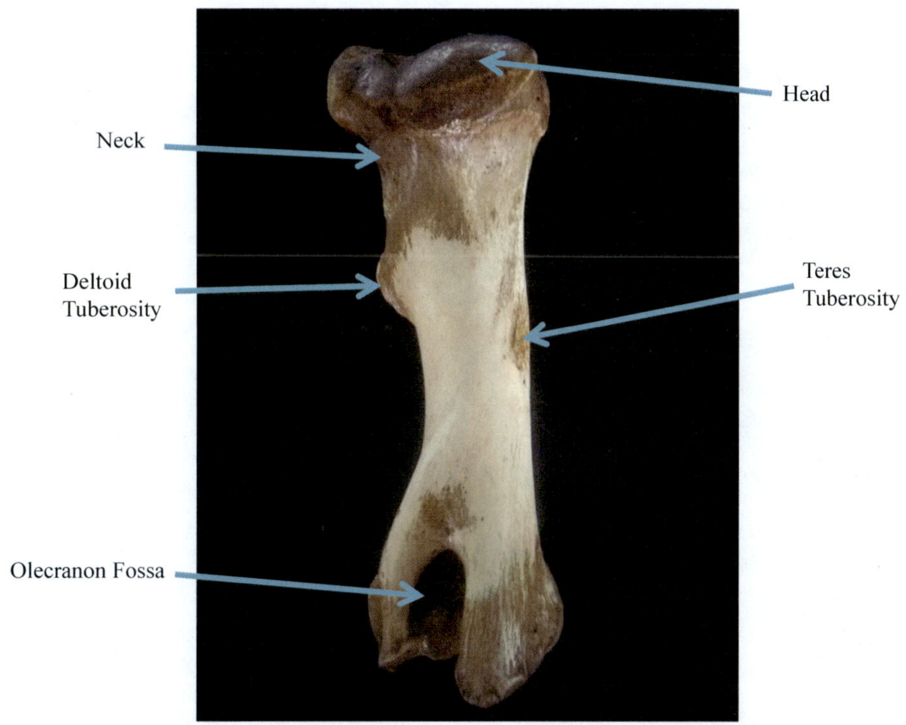

Humerus - Shaft (Muscular attachments on the shaft)

- Superficial pectoral muscle (Descending part) – inserts on the crest of humerus
- Deltoideus muscle – inserts on the deltoid tuberosity
- Brachialis muscle - which originates from the caudolateral surface and spirals around the bone (musculospiral groove)
- Medial and lateral heads of triceps brachii – originates from medial and lateral aspect of proximal aspect of the shaft of the humerus
- Coracobrachialis muscle – inserts on the medial surface of the humerus
- Teres major muscle – inserts on teres tuberosity

Humerus (Proximal Extremity)

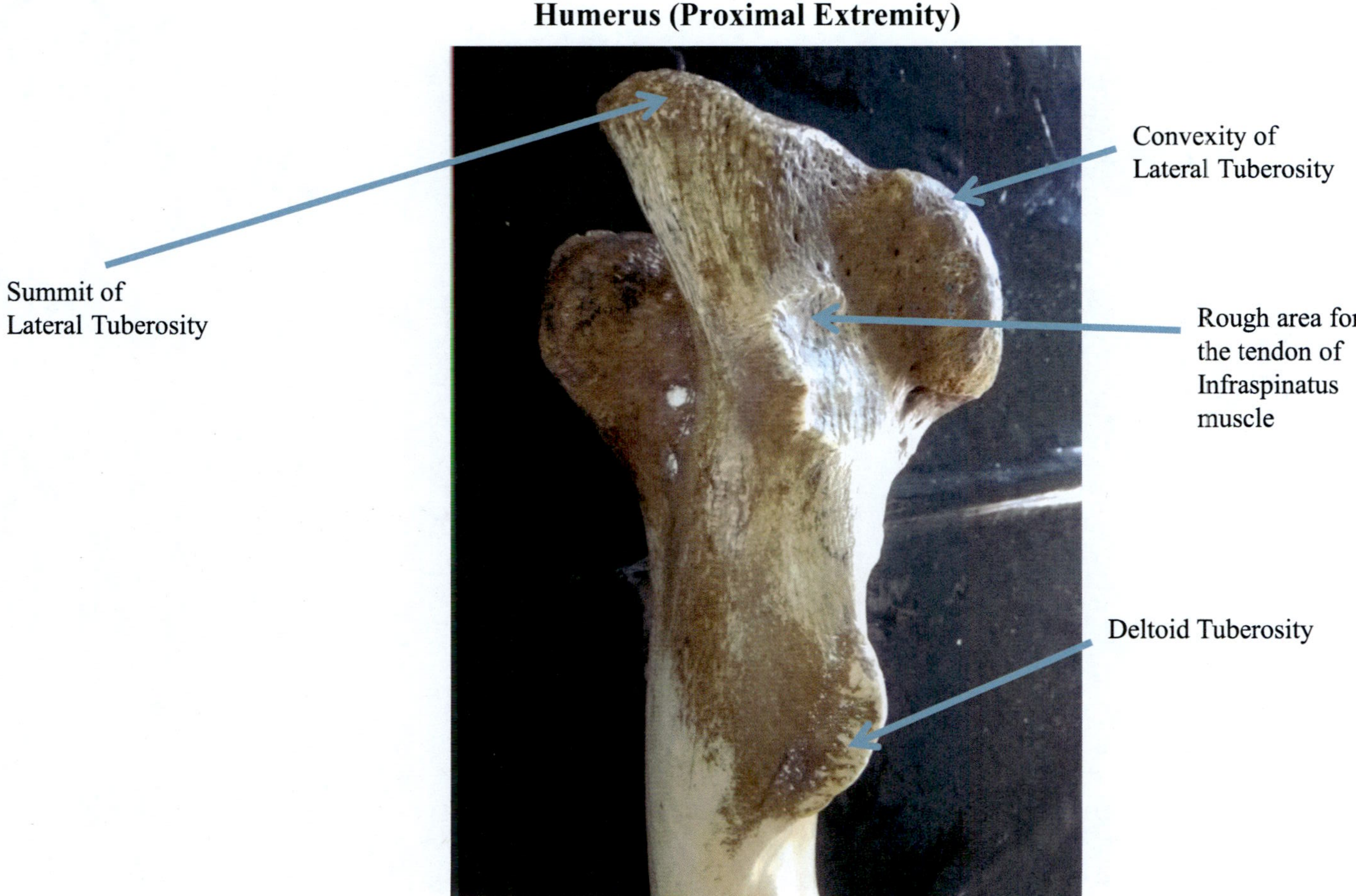

Humerus Distal End

At the distal extremity, the cranial surface contributes to the formation of the humeral condyle, which articulates with the radius and ulna at the elbow joint. This articulation allows for a wide range of motion in the forelimb, crucial for locomotion. The radial fossa is a depression on the cranial surface just proximal to the condyle, which accommodates the head of the radius during elbow flexion.

The lateral epicondyle is serves as a major origin point for craniolateral forearm muscles (extensors)

The medial epicondyle is serves as a major origin point for caudomedial forearm muscles (flexors)

Humerus (Medial Surface)

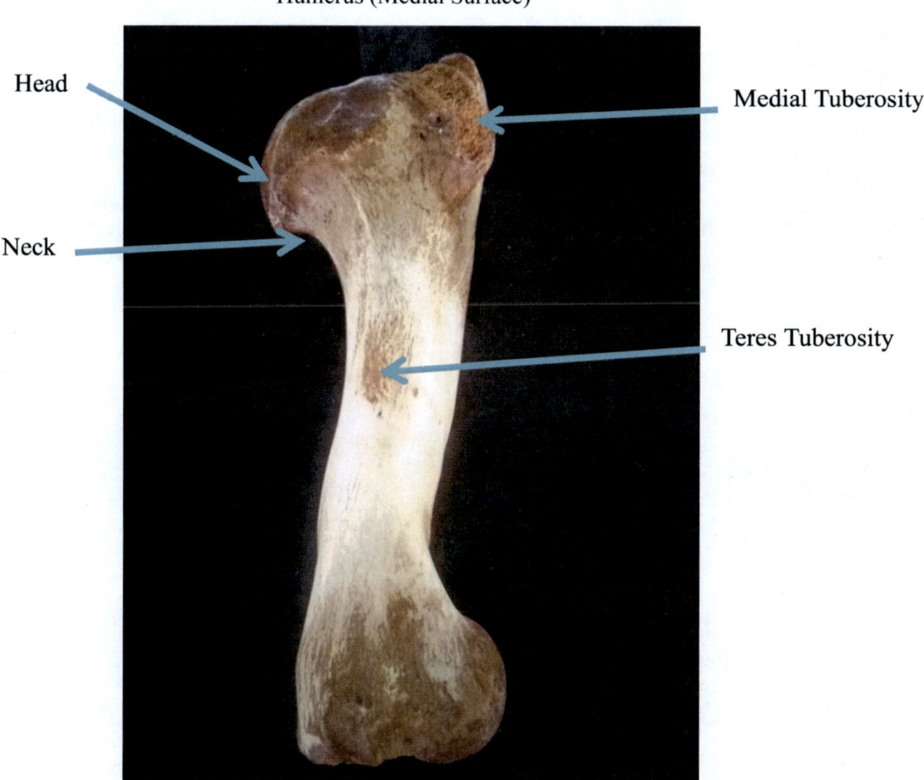

Major nerves that innervates the muscles of the arm region

Musculocutaneous nerve – it innervates coracobrachialis muscle, biceps brachii muscle and brachialis muscle.

Radial nerve – it innervates triceps brachii muscle and anconeus muscle.

Major blood vessels

Brachial artery – it gives blood supply to the muscle of the arm region.

Humerus (Lateral Surface)

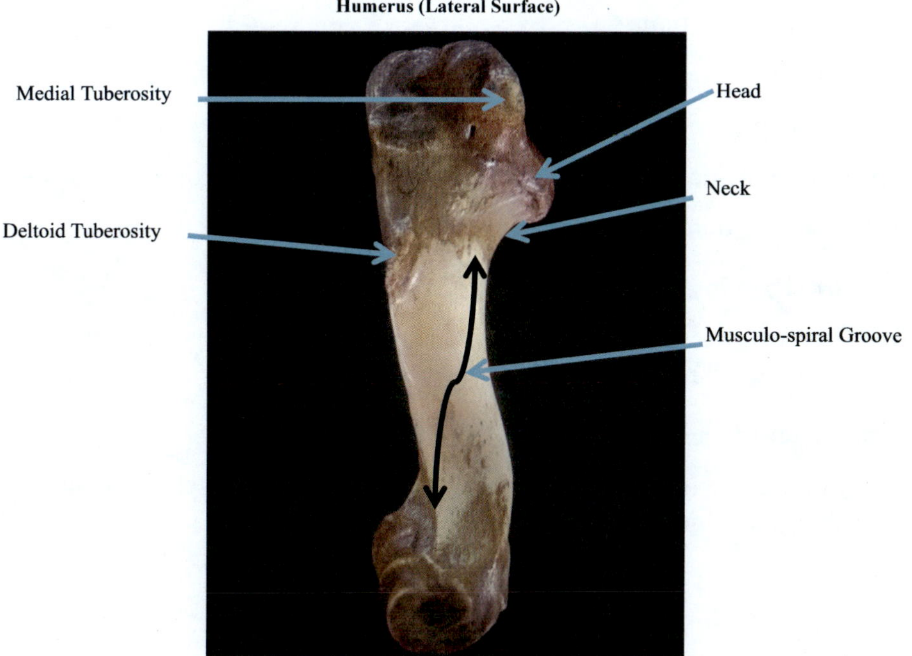

Humeral Fractures

Fractures due to trauma

- Complete fractures: The bone is broken all the way through.
- Incomplete fractures: Partial break, often seen in young calves.
- Comminuted fractures: The bone is shattered into multiple fragments.
- Spiral or oblique fractures are common in young animals.

Fractures during dystocia in young calves

- Physeal fractures: In young animals, fractures at the growth plates (epiphyseal regions).

Pathological Fractures

- Secondary to osteomyelitis or bone weakening diseases (e.g., calcium/ phosphorus imbalance, metabolic bone disease)

Humerus (Distal Extremity)

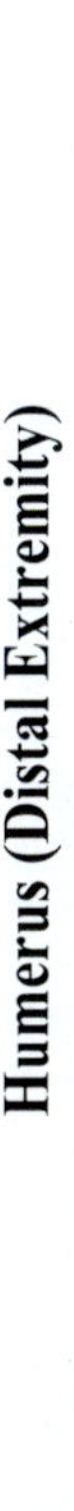

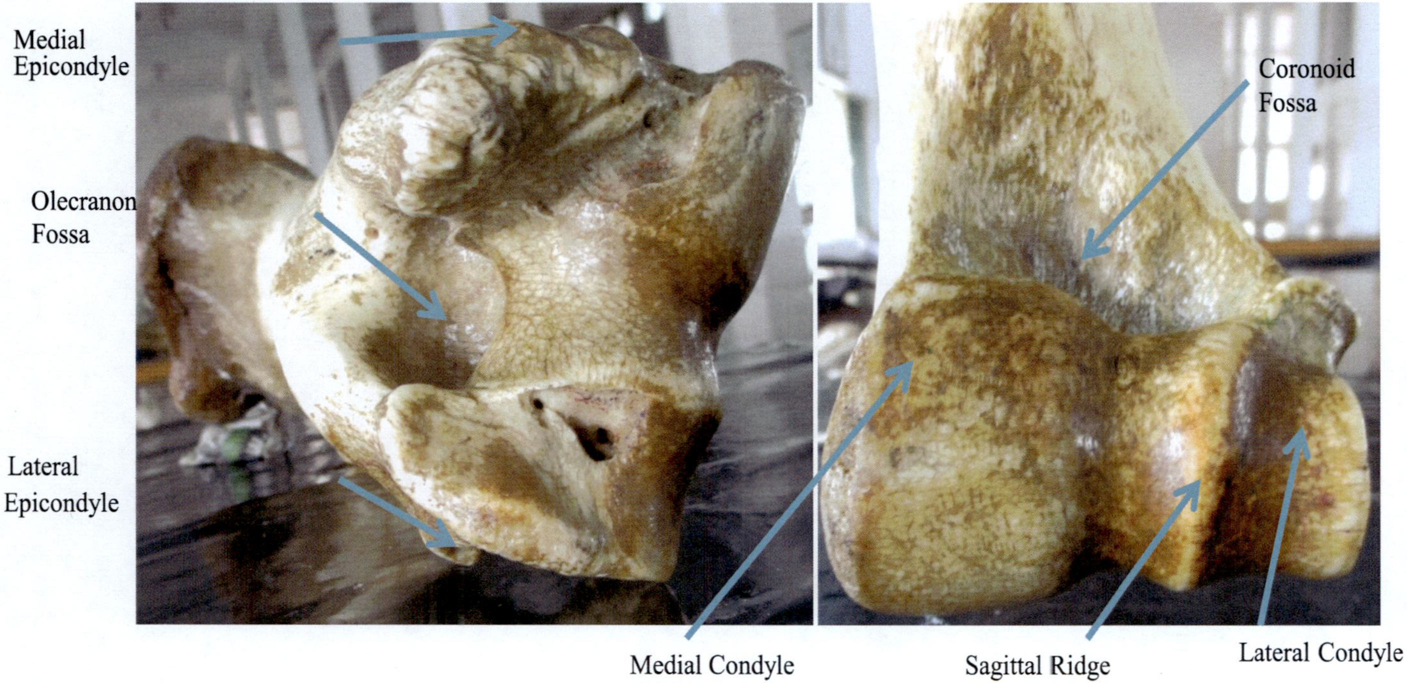

Nerve Injuries

1. Musculocutaneous Nerve Injury

Causes: Trauma to the shoulder or upper arm or compression injuries.

Clinical Signs: Inability to flex the elbow. Weakness when attempting to advance the forelimb. Reduced cutaneous sensation over the cranial aspect of the forearm.

2. Radial Nerve Injury (Medial aspect of the arm region)

Causes: trauma, prolonged recumbency, humeral fractures and improper restraint.

Clinical Signs

- Dropped elbow stance: The animal cannot extend the elbow, carpus, or digits.
- Knuckling at the fetlock joint due to flexor dominance.
- Non-weight bearing lameness.
- Muscle atrophy in chronic cases.

Radius

- **Two Surfaces**

  a) Cranial

  b) Caudal

- **Proximal Extremity**

  a) Lateral Articular Facet

  b) Medial Articular Facet

  c) Sagittal Cleft

  d) Coronoid Process

  e) Lateral Tuberosity

  f) Radial Tuberosity

  g) Medial Tuberosity

Distal Extremity of Radius and Ulna

- **Three Facets**

  a) Facet for Radial Carpal

  b) Facet for Intermediate Carpal

  c) Facet for Ulnar Carpal

Anatomy and Clinical Relevance

- The main weight-bearing bone of the forelimb.
- It is straight, robust, and located between the humerus (proximal) and the carpal bones (distal).

Ulna

- **Three parts**

  a) Olecranon Part

  b) Shaft

  c) Distal Extremity

- **Olecranon Part**

  a) Olecranon Process

  b) Anconeus Process

  c) Semilunar Notch

- **Distal Extremity**

  a) Styloid Process

- The olecranon process of the ulna is prominent and serves as the attachment site for the Tensor fascia antibrachii muscle and triceps brachii muscle, essential for weight-bearing and locomotion.

- The ulna is fused with the radius along most of its length, which is typical of ruminants.

- The fusion provides stability but limits rotational movement of the forelimb (e.g., pronation and supination)

Radius-Ulna (Cranio-lateral View)

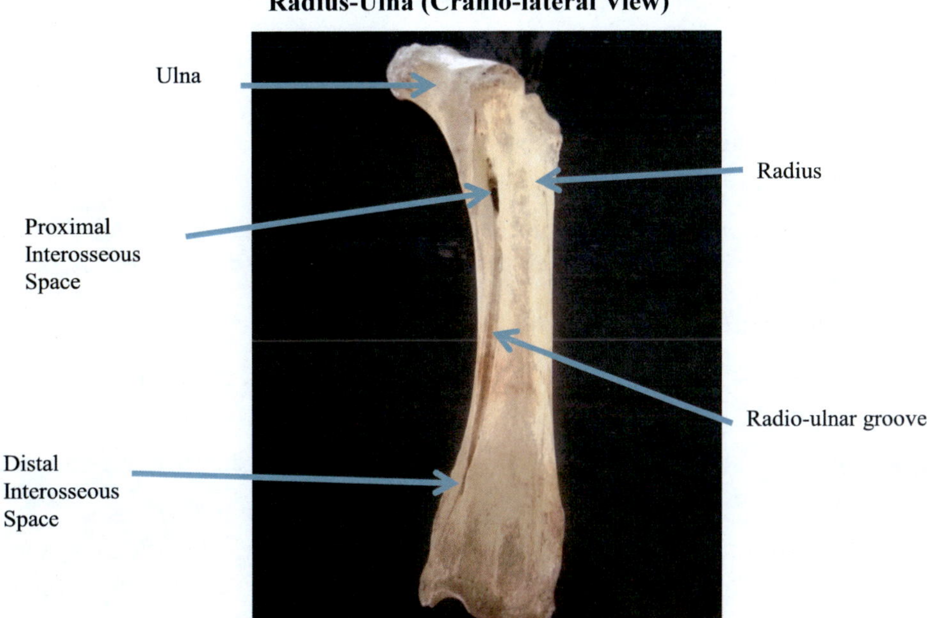

Key Palpable Landmarks – Radius and Ulna

- **Olecranon process:** Easily palpable and serves as a key landmark for evaluating elbow injuries.
- **Medial and lateral surfaces of the radius:** Useful for identifying swelling, fractures, or pain.

Together, the radius and ulna form the forearm and articulate proximally with the humerus at the elbow joint and distally with the carpal bones at the carpus.

Role of the Radius and Ulna in Locomotion

- The radius provides the primary support for the forelimb during weight-bearing.
- The ulna, although fused, plays a secondary role in stability and muscle attachment.
- The elbow joint (humeroradioulnar joint) allows for flexion and extension of the forelimb, which is crucial for movement and weight shifting.

Radius (Proximal Extremity)

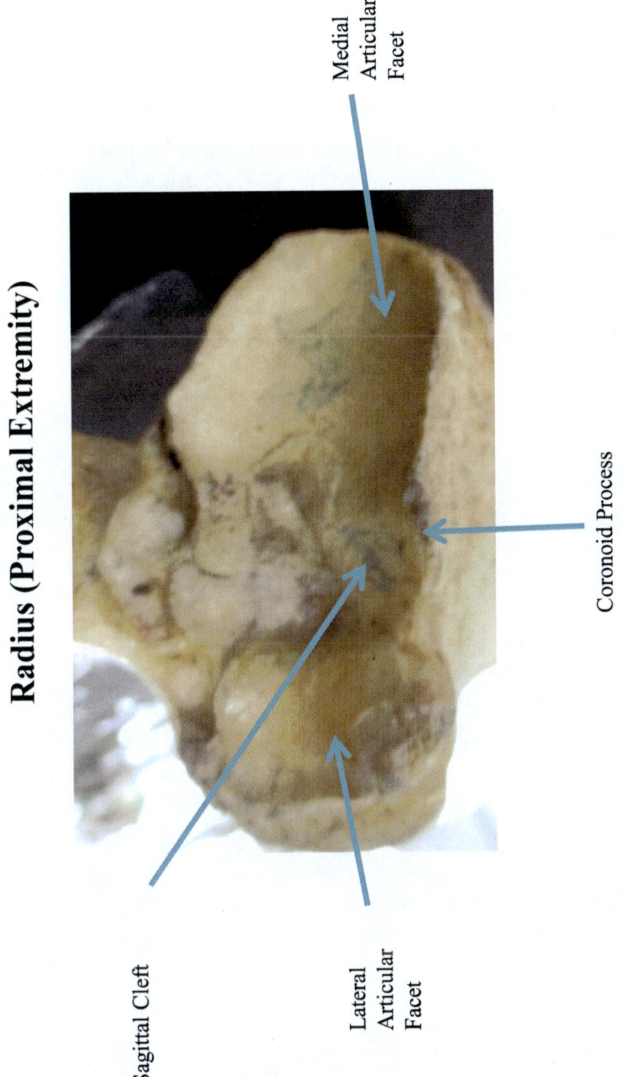

Muscle of forearm

Craniolateral forearm muscles: based on their action they are two types

1. **Extensor muscles:** Extensor carpi radialis, common digital extensor, medial digital extensor, lateral digital extensor and extensor carpi obliquus.
2. **Flexor muscles:** Ulnaris lateralis.

Caudomedial forearm muscles: based on their action they are flexor muscles

1. **Superficial Group Flexors:** Pronator teres (vestigial), flexor carpi radialis and flexor carpi ulnaris.
2. **Deep Group Flexors:** Superficial digital flexor and deep digital flexor.

Major nerves of forearm: Radial nerve, median nerve and ulnar nerve.

Major blood vessel in the forearm: Median artery and radial artery.

Radius-Ulna (Proximal Extremity)

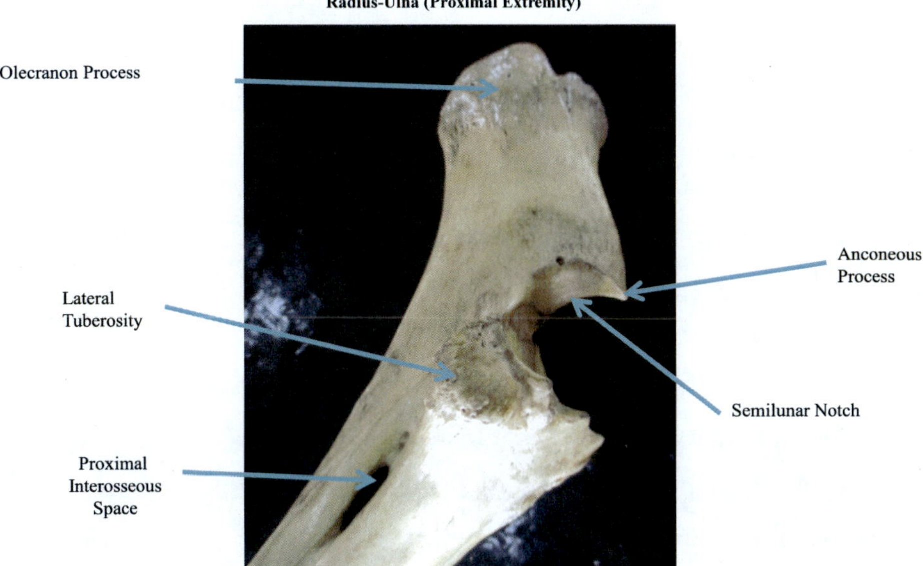

Fractures of the Radius and Ulna

Common Causes

- Trauma: Falls, kicks, or collisions with heavy equipment.
- Radial fractures and olecranon fractures are commonly seen in cattle due to trauma
- Calves may suffer fractures due to being trampled or during assisted calving.

Fracture Types

- **Transverse fractures:** Straight break across the bone.
- **Oblique fractures:** Diagonal fracture line.
- **Comminuted fractures:** Bone shattered into multiple pieces.
- **Open fractures:** Fractures with overlying skin damage, leading to increased risk of infection.

Radius (Cranial View)

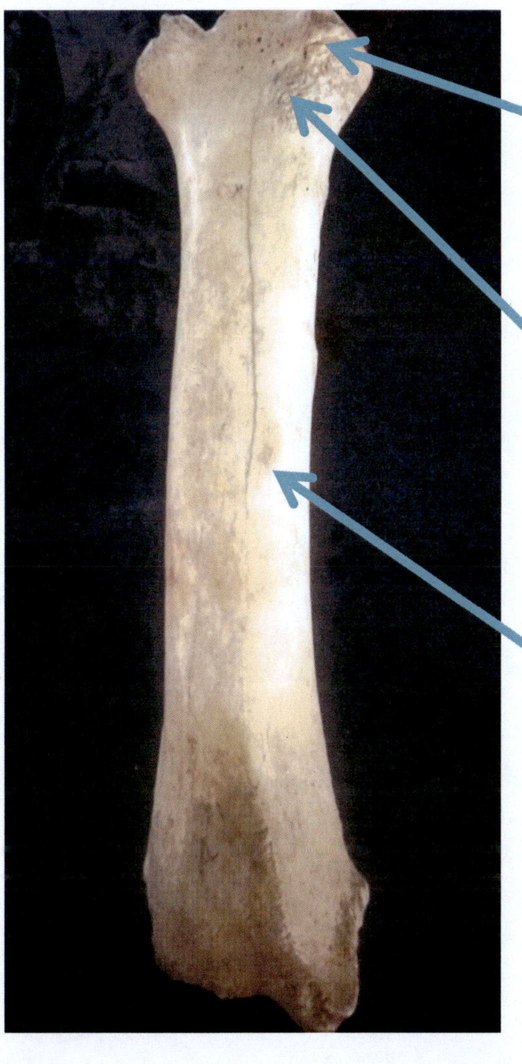

Clinical condition related to ulna

Olecranon Bursitis ("Shoe Boil")

Cause: Repeated trauma or pressure over the olecranon process of the ulna, often due to lying on hard surfaces.

Clinical Signs: Swelling over the elbow (fluid-filled bursa). Mild to moderate lameness in severe cases.

Radius-Ulna (Cranio-Lateral View)

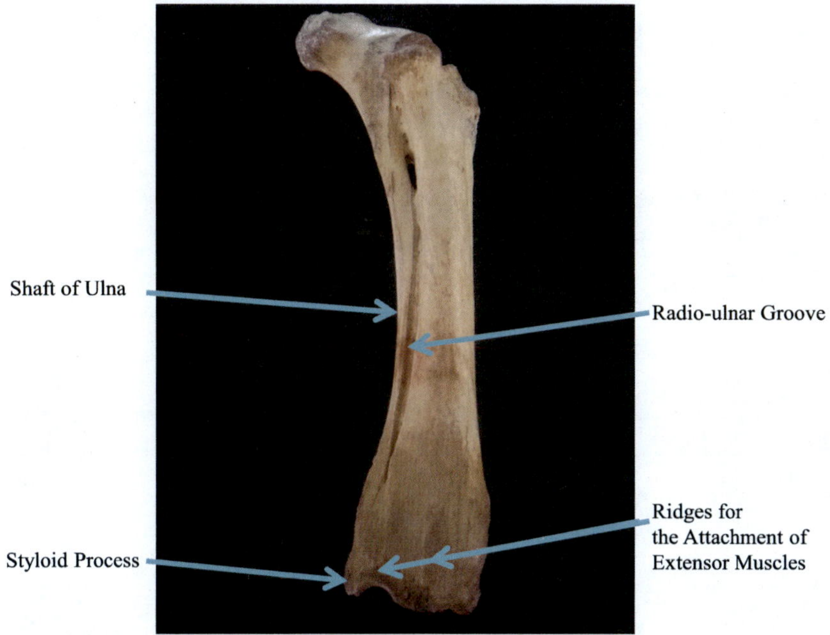

Radial Nerve Injury

Cause: Injury to the radial nerve can occur at the craniolateral side of the radius and ulna, often from trauma, prolonged recumbency, or improper restraint.

Clinical Signs

- Dropped elbow stance due to inability to extend the elbow.
- Knuckling of the fetlock.
- Non-weight bearing on the affected limb.

Radius-Ulna (Distal Extremity)

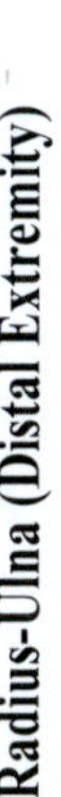

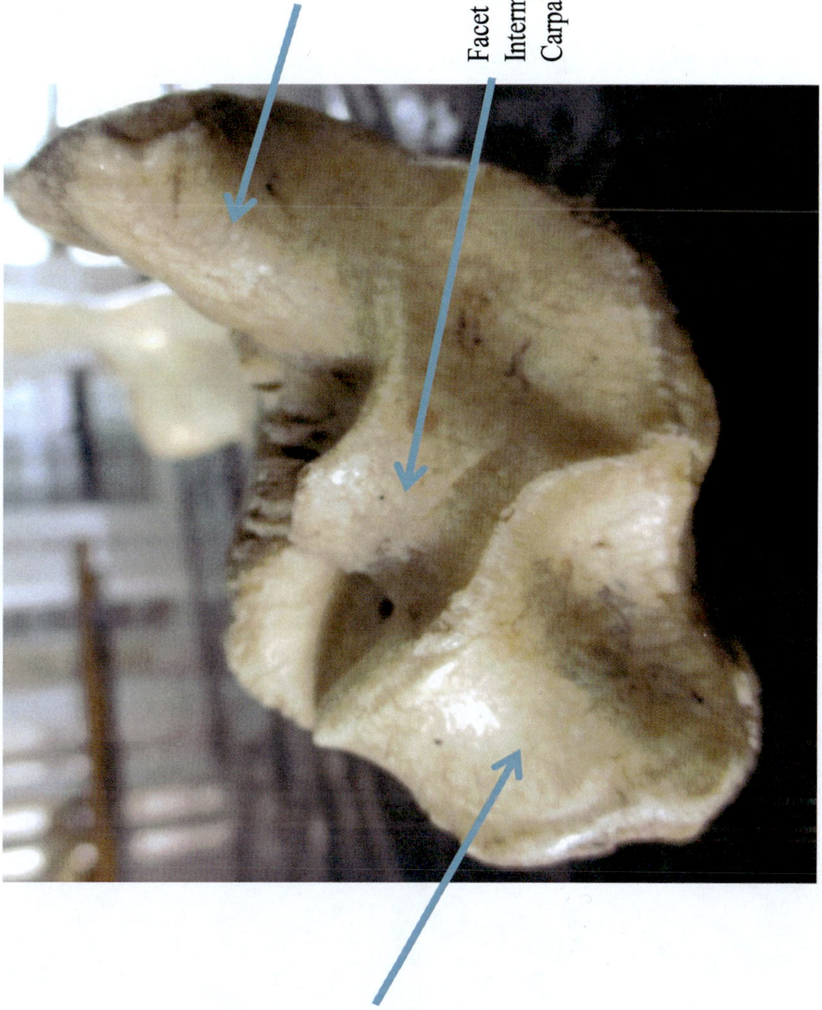

Angular Limb Deformities

Angular deformities are very common in young calves, often they lead to lameness.

Cause

- Abnormal growth of the distal radial growth plate in young calves.
- Nutritional deficiencies (e.g., vitamin D, calcium, phosphorus).
- Trauma or infection affecting the growth plate.

Clinical Signs

- Varus deformity: Medial deviation of the limb.
- Valgus deformity: Lateral deviation of the limb.

Osteomyelitis

- Osteomyelitis is a complex and challenging condition seen across all species, characterized by inflammation and infection of the bone and bone marrow.
- In young animals, Salmonella species—particularly the cattle-adapted Salmonella Dublin—are frequently associated with clinical disease.
- In older animals, Trueperella pyogenes is the most commonly isolated pathogen, often found in combination with anaerobes such as Fusobacterium necrophorum.
- In neonatal animals, osteomyelitis may also develop secondary to fractures of the metacarpus or metatarsus, particularly following the improper use of calving chains during dystocia.
- Actinomycosis—commonly known as "lumpy jaw"—is a specific form of osteomyelitis that affects the mandible and sometimes the maxilla in cattle.

Carpals

- **Arranged in Two Rows**
  a) Proximal
  b) Distal
- **Proximal Row**
  a) Radial
  b) Intermediate
  c) Ulnar
  d) Accessory
- **Distal Row**
  a) Fused 2nd and 3rd
  b) 4th

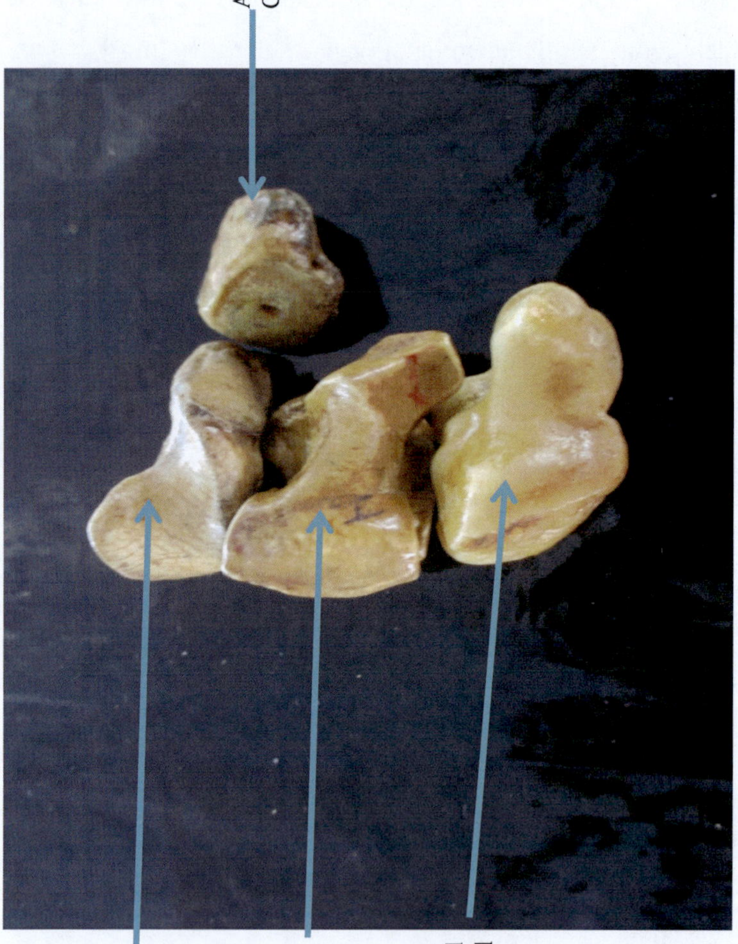

Carpals of Proximal Row

Accessory Carpal

Ulnar Carpal

Intermediate Carpal

Radial Carpal

Proximal Row

1. Radial Carpal Bone

- Location: Medial bone in the proximal row.
- Articulations:
  - Proximally with the radius.
  - Distally with the second and third carpal bones.
- Function: Provides support and stability to the medial side of the carpal joint.
- Clinical Note: Fractures or injuries to this bone can compromise weight-bearing capacity.

2. Intermediate Carpal Bone

- Location: Positioned between the radial and ulnar carpal bones.
- Articulations:
  - Proximally with the radius.
  - Distally with the third carpal bone.
- Function: Acts as a central stabilizer, transmitting forces evenly across the carpus.
- Clinical Note: Injuries can lead to uneven load distribution and joint instability.

Carpals of Distal Row

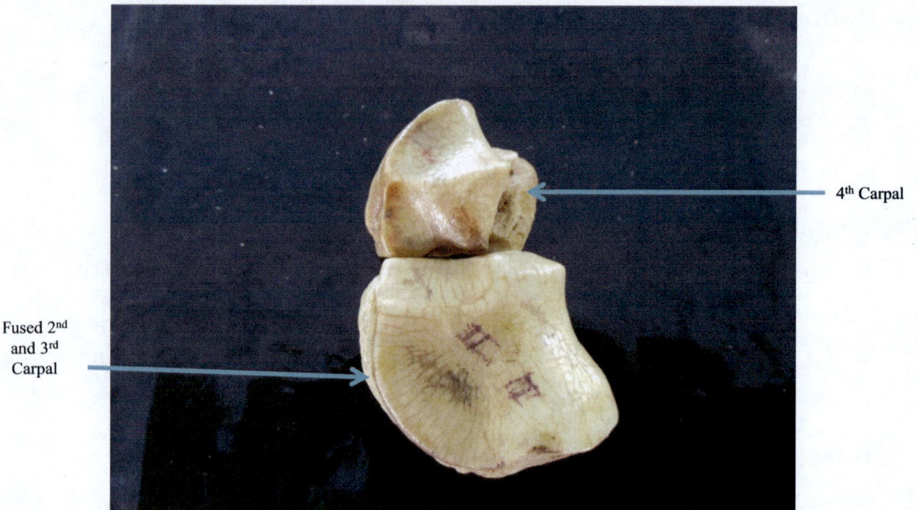

3. Ulnar Carpal Bone

- **Location:** Lateral bone in the proximal row.
- **Articulations:**
  - Proximally with the ulna (if present as a vestige).
  - Distally with the fourth carpal bone.
- **Function:** Provides lateral support to the carpal joint.
- **Clinical Note:** Subject to stress injuries due to its positioning in weight-bearing and lateral stabilization.

4. Accessory Carpal Bone

- **Location:** Palmar and lateral to the ulnar carpal bone.
- **Articulations:**
  - Proximally with the ulnar carpal bone.
- **Function:**
  - Acts as an anchor for the flexor carpi ulnaris and ulnaris lateralis tendons.
  - Provides leverage for flexor tendons.
- **Clinical Note:** Commonly involved in trauma or inflammation (e.g., carpal hygroma).

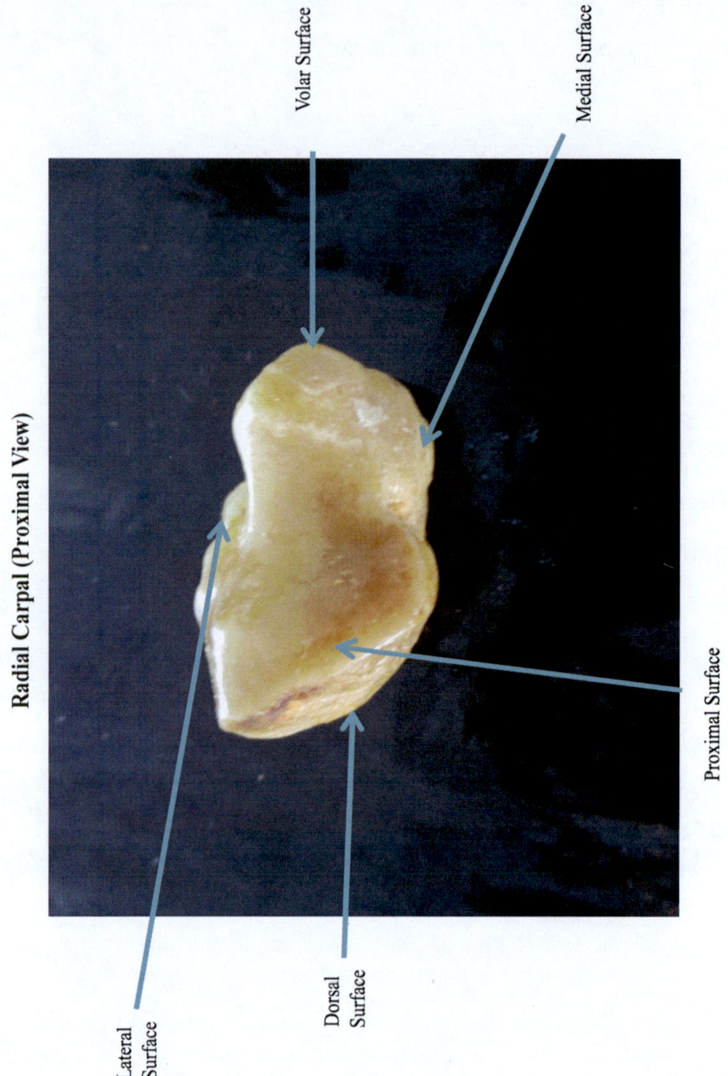

Radial Carpal (Proximal View)

Distal Row

1. Fused Second and Third Carpal Bone

- **Location**
  - Proximally with the radial and intermediate carpal bones.
  - Distally with the third metacarpal bone (major weight-bearing metacarpal).
- **Function**
  - Bears significant weight.
  - Transmits forces from the proximal row to the metacarpus.
- **Clinical Note:** Prone to fractures due to its weight-bearing role.

2. Fourth Carpal Bone

- **Location:** Lateral bone in the distal row.
- **Articulations:**
  - Proximally with the ulnar carpal bone.
  - Distally with the third and fourth metacarpal bones.
- **Function:** Provides lateral stability and shares the load with the third carpal bone.
- **Clinical Note:** May be involved in trauma-related injuries, especially in cases of lateral stress.

Radial Carpal (Distal View)

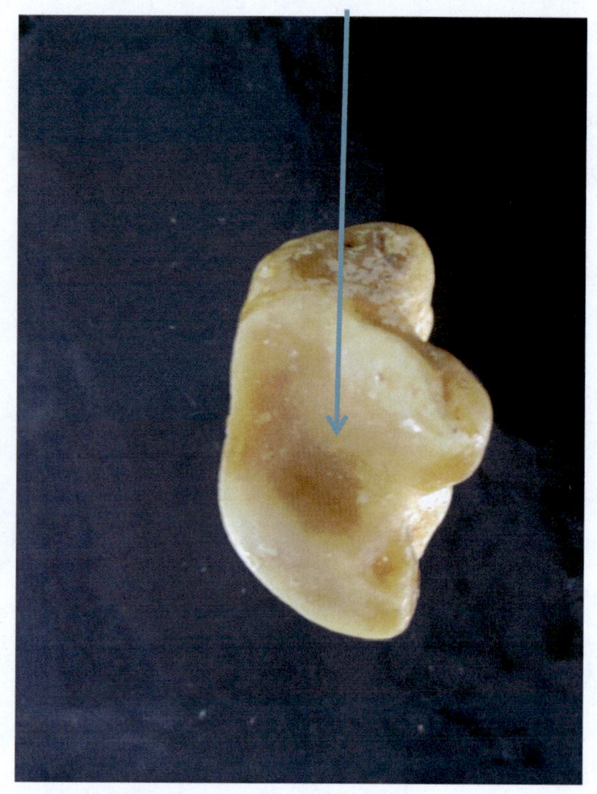

Joints of the Carpus

The carpal bones are connected by synovial joints, which are highly significant for mobility:

1. Antebrachiocarpal Joint

- Between the radius and ulna (proximally) and the proximal row of carpal bones.
- Greatest range of motion.

2. Middle Carpal Joint

- Between the proximal and distal rows of carpal bones.
- Moderate range of motion.

3. Carpometacarpal Joint

- Between the distal row of carpal bones and the metacarpals.
- Minimal motion.

Each joint is supported by a joint capsule and collateral ligaments.

Intermediate Carpal (Proximal View)

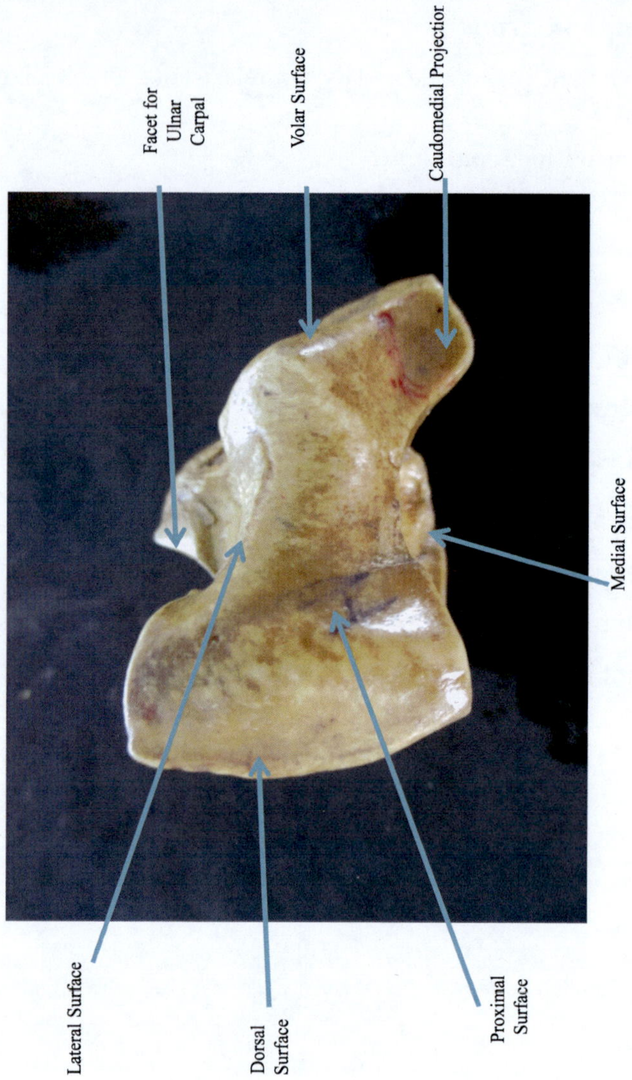

Facet for Ulnar Carpal

Volar Surface

Caudomedial Projectior

Medial Surface

Lateral Surface

Dorsal Surface

Proximal Surface

Tendons associated with the carpals

1. Flexor Tendons (Palmar Aspect)

- **Superficial Digital Flexor Tendon (SDFT):** Attaches to the second phalanx, aiding in flexion.
- **Deep Digital Flexor Tendon (DDFT):** Attaches to the third phalanx, providing additional flexion and support.
- **Flexor Retinaculum:** A fibrous sheath that secures the flexor tendons in place.

2. Extensor Tendons (Dorsal Aspect)

- **Common Digital Extensor Tendon:** Extends to the digits and facilitates extension.
- **Lateral Digital Extensor Tendon:** Assists in extending the digits.

3. Other Tendons

- **Ulnaris Lateralis:** Contributes to lateral stability and flexion.
- **Flexor Carpi Radialis:** Helps in flexing the carpus.

Intermediate Carpal (Distal View)

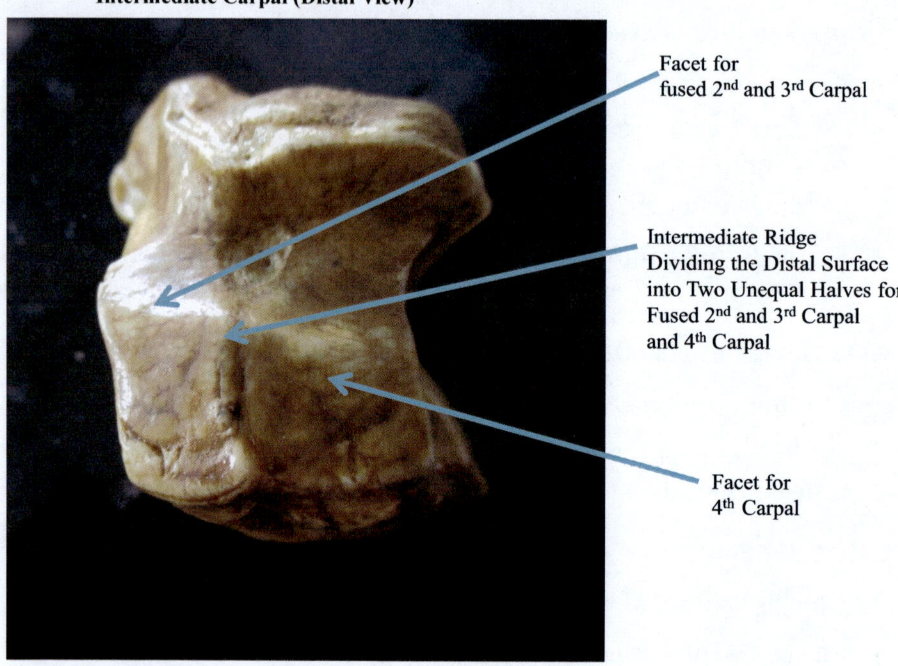

Nerves of carpal region

The carpal region is innervated by the brachial plexus:

Median Nerve: Innervates the tendons of flexor muscles. Supplies the palmar aspect of the carpus and digits.

Ulnar Nerve: Provides motor innervation to tendons of some flexor muscles (e.g., flexor carpi ulnaris). Supplies sensory innervation to the lateral carpal and digital areas.

Radial Nerve: Innervates the tendons of extensor muscles (e.g., common digital extensor, extensor carpi radialis). Supplies sensory input to the dorsal aspect of the carpus.

Ulnar Carpal (Proximal View)

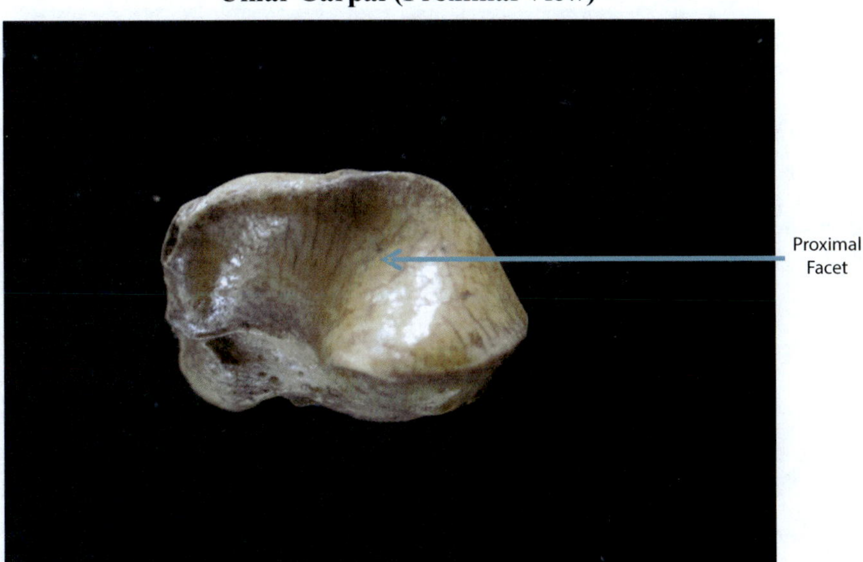

Blood Vessels of carpal region

The carpal region is richly vascularized, with the following key arteries and veins:

Median Artery: The main blood supply to the carpal region, passing distally to the digits.

Branches into the palmar arteries.

Radial Artery: Supplies the medial aspect of the carpus.

Ulnar Artery: Supplies the lateral aspect of the carpus.

Venous Drainage: Accomplished by the cephalic vein and accessory cephalic vein, which drain into the larger venous system.

Accessory Carpal

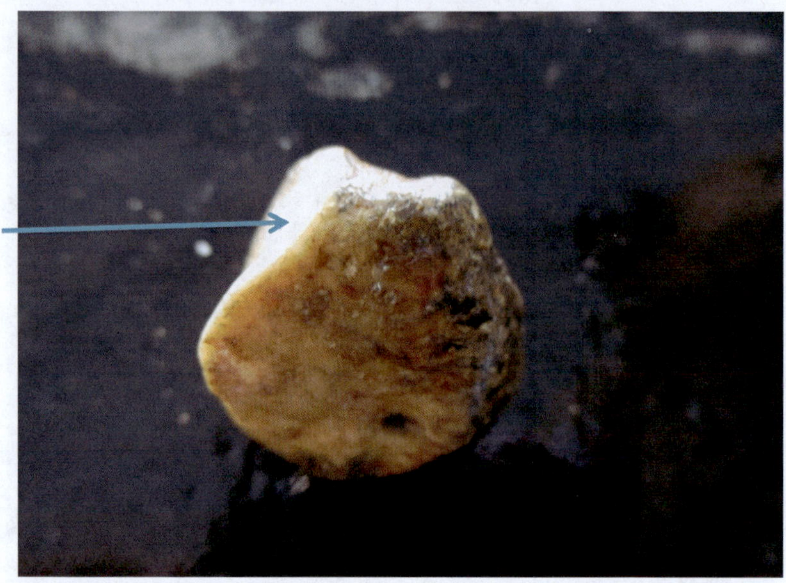

Trauma and Fractures – carpus region

- Carpal fractures in cattle, though less frequent than metacarpal or metatarsal fractures, do occur and are typically managed using external coaptation or cast immobilization. The decision to pursue treatment—and its likelihood of success—depends on several factors, including the fracture's type and location, the cost of care, and the animal's economic value.
- Carpal fractures are relatively common in cattle due to falls, excessive force during movement, or handling.
- The radial carpal bone and third carpal bone are more susceptible to fractures due to their weight-bearing role.
- Fractures can lead to lameness, swelling, and reluctance to move.

Fused 2nd and 3rd Carpal (Proximal View)

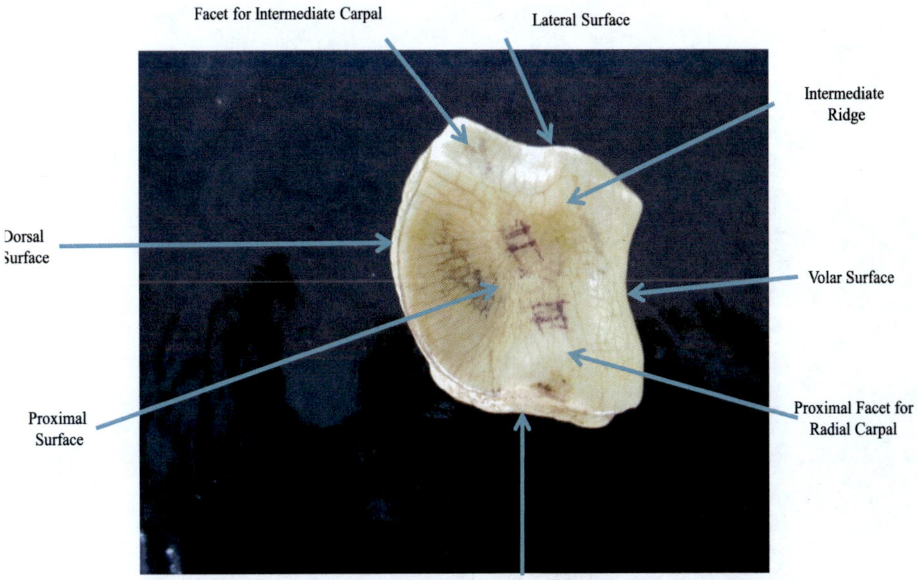

Carpal Hygroma: Clinical condition

- Carpal Hygroma is a localized, firm swelling of the soft tissues, often fluctuant and typically non-painful, located over the dorsal aspect of the carpus. In some cases, the swelling may be surrounded by fibrous tissue and contain purulent material. This condition is commonly seen in bovines due to their tendency to rest or rise by placing pressure on their carpal joints first.
- **Causes:** Carpal hygroma usually results from repetitive trauma or pressure over bony prominences, particularly at weight-bearing points. It can also develop secondary to a subcutaneous hematoma. In rare cases, it may be congenital or associated with Brucellosis infection.
- **Clinical Signs:** Soft, fluid-filled swelling located subcutaneously, commonly over the carpus or tarsus, typically painless, no associated lameness and swelling may vary in consistency depending on chronicity or secondary infection

Fused 2nd and 3rd Carpal (Distal View)

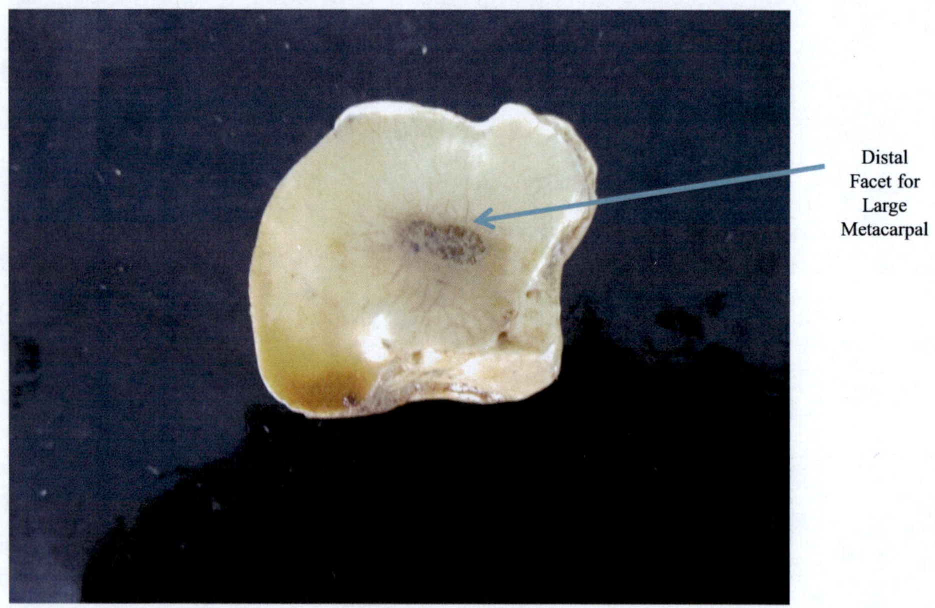

Tendon and Ligament Injuries – carpus region

- The flexor retinaculum and associated tendons are closely related to the carpal bones. In cattle, the flexor retinaculum is a robust fibrous band that forms the roof of the carpal canal, a tunnel that accommodates the flexor tendons of the forelimb. This structure helps to stabilize the tendons during movement. Additionally, the carpal canal in cattle also contains the median nerve, with the flexor retinaculum being an integral part of it.
- Trauma or excessive strain can lead to tenosynovitis or rupture of supporting structures in the carpal region.

4th Carpal (Proximal View)

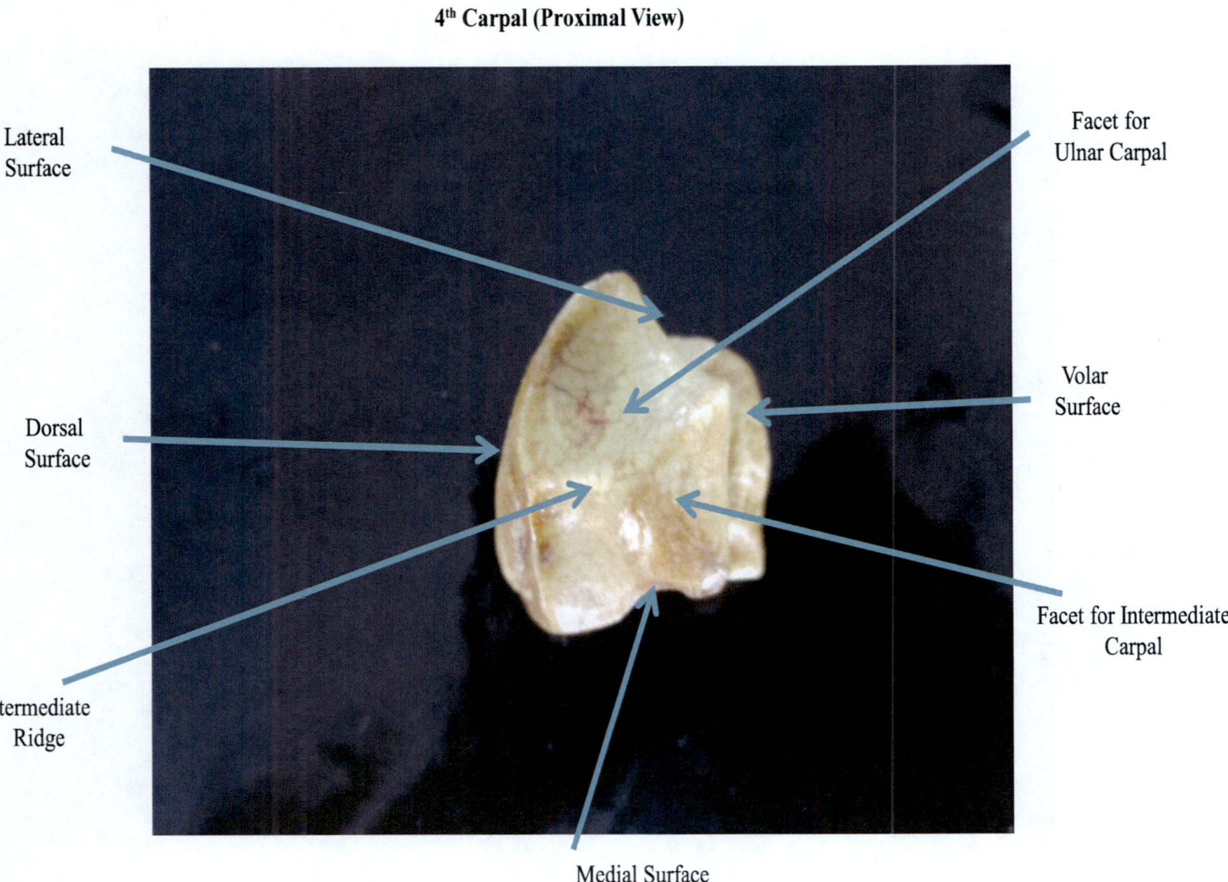

Carpitis (Arthritis of the Carpal Joint)

- Carpitis, or arthritis of the carpal joint, in cattle can occur due to trauma, infection, or degenerative changes. Typical symptoms include pain during flexion, bony remodeling, and swelling of the carpal joint.
- Treatment options may include the removal of loose bone fragments, repair of cartilage damage, and in more severe cases, surgical fusion (arthrodesis) of the carpal joints.

Causes

- Trauma or chronic stress.
- Joint infections (e.g., hematogenous spread in calves).
- Degenerative joint disease (DJD).

4th Carpal (Distal View)

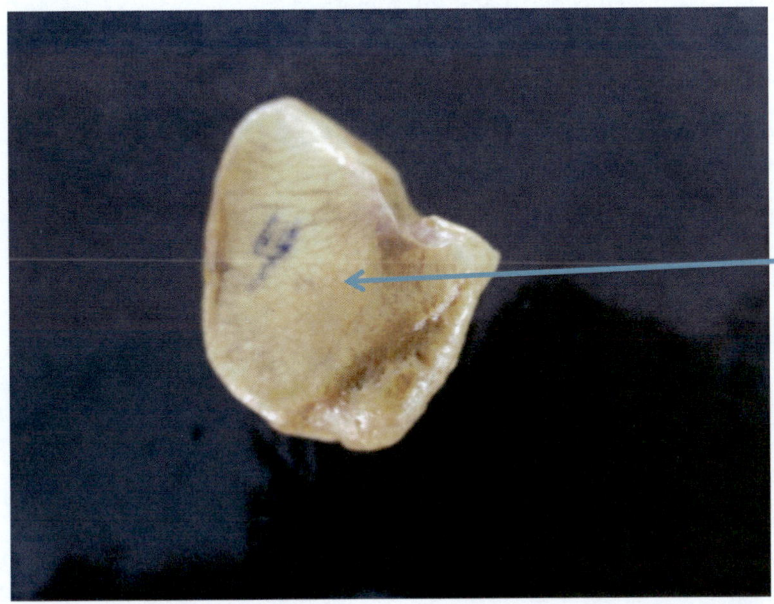

Carpal Canal Syndrome

- Carpal tunnel syndrome (CTS) is a condition caused by nerve compression in the wrist, most commonly observed in humans.
- Though rarer, it has also been reported in animals such as horses, dogs, and cats, but is less frequently seen in cattle.
- In animals, CTS symptoms may include pain, numbness, and weakness in the affected limb. These animals might show signs of discomfort, such as reluctance to move the affected limb, pain, or changes in their gait.
- Diagnostic and treatment methods for CTS in animals can differ from those used in humans.

Metacarpal

- Large metacarpal (fused 3rd and 4th metacarpal)
- Small metacarpal (5th metacarpal)

Large Metacarpal

- **Two Surfaces**

  a) Dorsal

  b) Volar

- **Dorsal Surface**

  a) Metacarpal Tuberosity

  b) Dorsal Vascular Groove

  c) Proximal Interosseous Foramen

  d) Distal Interosseous Foramen

- **Volar Surface**

  a) Volar Vascular Groove

  b) Proximal Interosseous Foramen

  c) Distal Interosseous Foramen

  d) Facet for Attachment of Small Metacarpal (5th) near lateral border

Large Metacarpal

- **Two borders**

  a) Medial

  b) Lateral

- **Proximal Extremity**

  a) Facet for 2nd and 3rd Fused Carpals

  b) Facet for 4th Carpal

- **Distal Extremity**

  a) Lateral Condyle

  b) Medial Condyle

c) Sagittal Ridge

d) Sagittal Notch

I. Fused Metacarpals (Metacarpal III and IV)

The Metacarpal III and IV are fused into a single bony structure, forming the cannon bone.

A longitudinal groove on the dorsal and palmar surfaces of the cannon bone indicates the fusion line.

Special Features

Proximal End: Articulates with the distal row of carpal bones. Contains grooves and ridges for ligament and tendon attachments.

Distal End: Forms the fetlock joints with the proximal phalanges. Equipped with two condyles (medial and lateral) for articulation with the digits.

II. Vestigial Metacarpals

Second Metacarpal (Mc II) and Fifth Metacarpal (Mc V) are vestigial or absent.

These remnants do not play a significant role in weight-bearing or locomotion.

Metacarpal (Dorsal View)

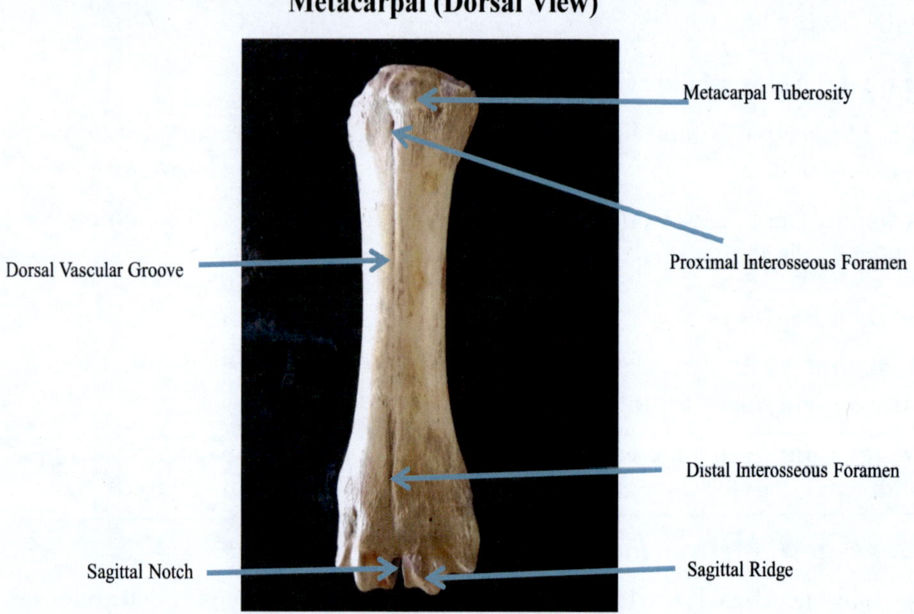

Associated Structures of Metacarpals

Joints

Carpometacarpal Joint: Between the distal carpal bones and the metacarpals.

Metacarpophalangeal Joints (Fetlock Joints): Between the distal metacarpal condyles and the proximal phalanges.

Tendons

Extensor Tendons (Dorsal Aspect):

Common Digital Extensor: Attaches to both digits and extends them.

Lateral Digital Extensor: Attaches to the lateral digit.

Flexor Tendons (Palmar Aspect):

Superficial Digital Flexor: Binds to the proximal phalanges for flexion.

Deep Digital Flexor: Extends to the distal phalanges for flexion.

Metacarpal (Volar View)

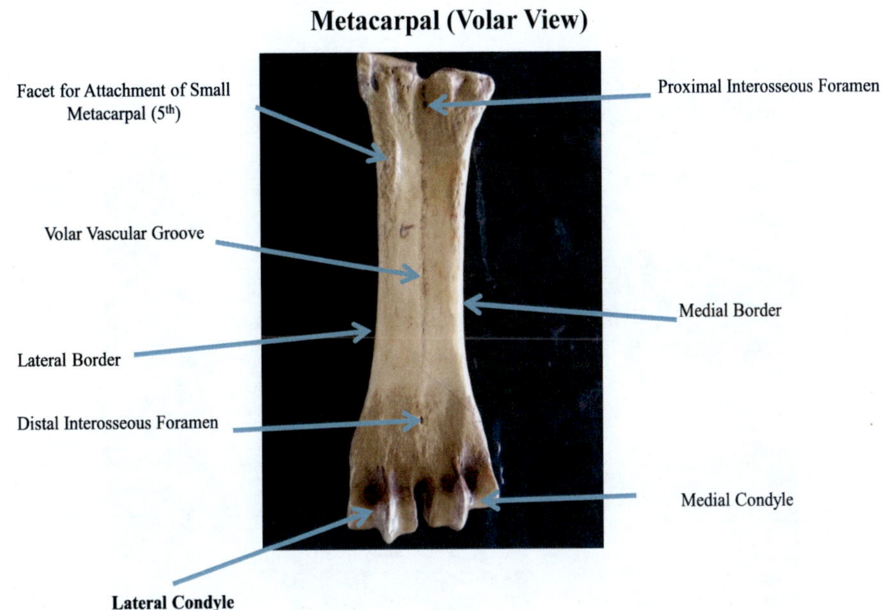

Associated Structures of Metacarpals

Ligaments

Interosseous Ligament: Between the fused Mc III and Mc IV, supporting structural integrity.

Collateral Ligaments: Stabilize the fetlock joints.

Blood Supply and Innervation

Blood supply from the median artery and its branches.

Nerve supply from the median, ulnar, and radial nerves.

Metacarpal (Proximal Extremity)

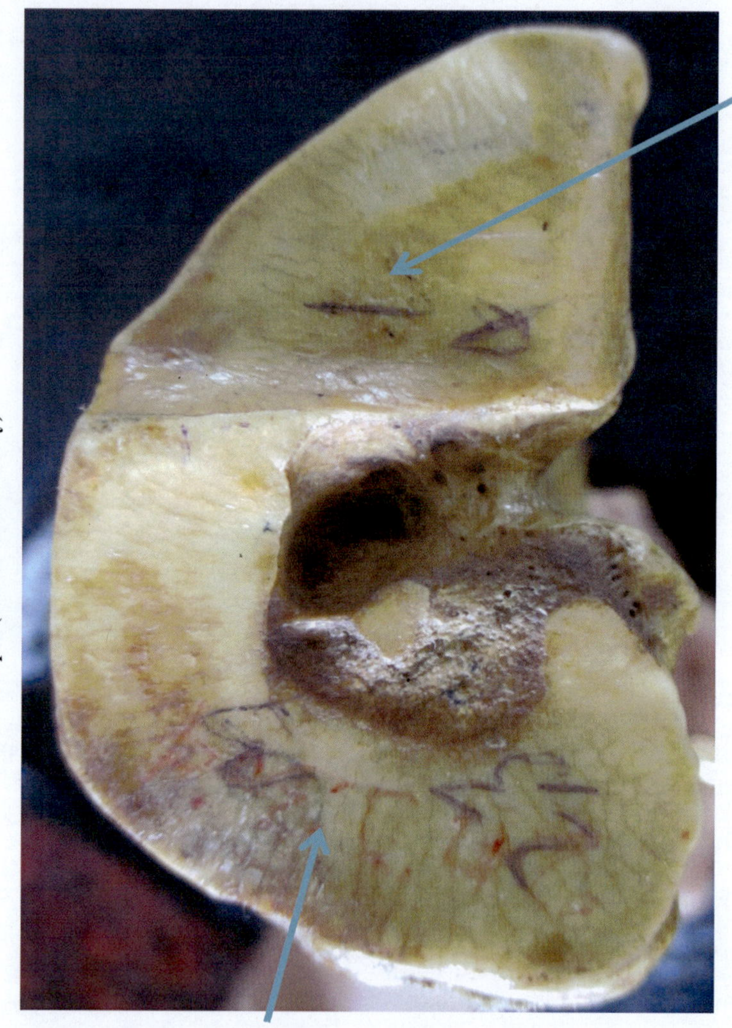

Clinical Significance of metacarpals

1. Fractures

Midshaft fractures are most frequent, commonly caused by trauma (e.g., falls, accidents).

Stress Fractures: Can occur due to repetitive strain, especially in athletic or working cattle.

Clinical Signs: Swelling, pain on palpation, and lameness.

2. Osteomyelitis

Infection of the metacarpal bone due to open fractures, penetrating wounds, or systemic infections.

Presents with swelling, heat, and lameness.

3. Metacarpal Periostitis:

Inflammation of the periosteum due to repetitive trauma or excessive strain.

Localized swelling along the metacarpal groove.

4. Angular Limb Deformities

Congenital or acquired deformities, such as valgus (outward deviation) or varus (inward deviation) of the metacarpal bones.

Clinical Significance of metacarpals

5. Tendon and Ligament Injuries

Overuse or trauma can lead to injuries in the extensor or flexor tendons and associated ligaments.

Common in cattle subjected to high mechanical loads.

6. Arthritis or Joint Disorders

Involving the fetlock joint due to trauma, infection, or age-related wear.

7. Developmental Abnormalities

In young calves, improper development of the metacarpals can lead to structural issues affecting gait and weight distribution.

8. Nerve and Blood Vessel Damage

Injuries to the metacarpal region can damage overlying nerves or blood vessels, resulting in impaired mobility or ischemia of the digits.

Digits and Phalanges

- **Two Digits**
- **Each Digit has three Phalanges**

  a) First Phalanx

  b) Second Phalanx

  c) Third Phalanx

Digits with Phalanges (Dorsal View)

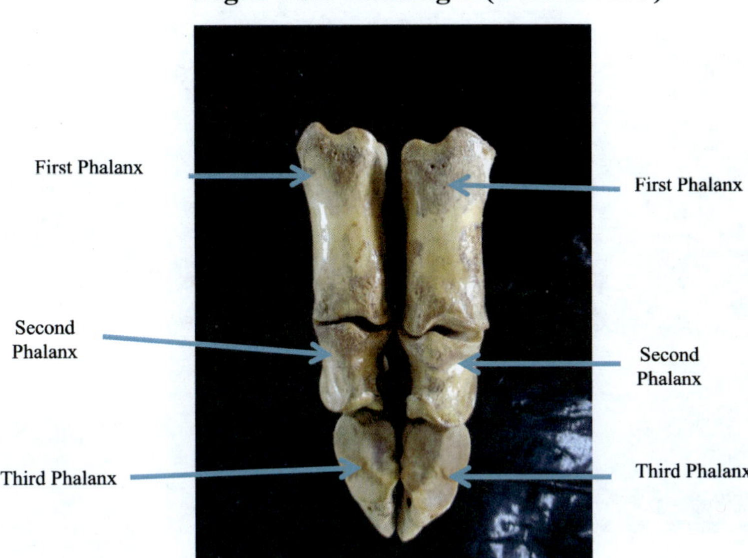

The digits and phalanges of cattle are critical for locomotion, weight-bearing, and providing stability. Since cattle are cloven-hoofed animals, their digits are divided into two functional weight-bearing digits on each limb, supported by phalanges, joints, and associated structures.

Digits

1. **Functional Digits:** Third Digit (Medial claw): Medial and weight-bearing. Fourth Digit (Lateral claw): Lateral and weight-bearing. Together, they form the cloven hoof.
2. **Vestigial Digits:** Second and Fifth Digits, represented by small bony remnants called dewclaws, located on the back of the fetlock joint. These do not play a role in weight-bearing or locomotion.

Phalanges: Each functional digit consists of three phalanges:

1. **Proximal Phalanx (P1):** Also called the long pastern bone. Articulates proximally with the metacarpals and distally with the middle phalanx.
2. **Middle Phalanx (P2):** Also called the short pastern bone. Articulates proximally with the proximal phalanx and distally with the distal phalanx.
3. **Distal Phalanx (P3):** Also called the coffin bone. Enclosed within the hoof capsule and has a crescent-shaped distal border. Anchors the deep digital flexor tendon.

First Phalanx (Proximal Extremity)

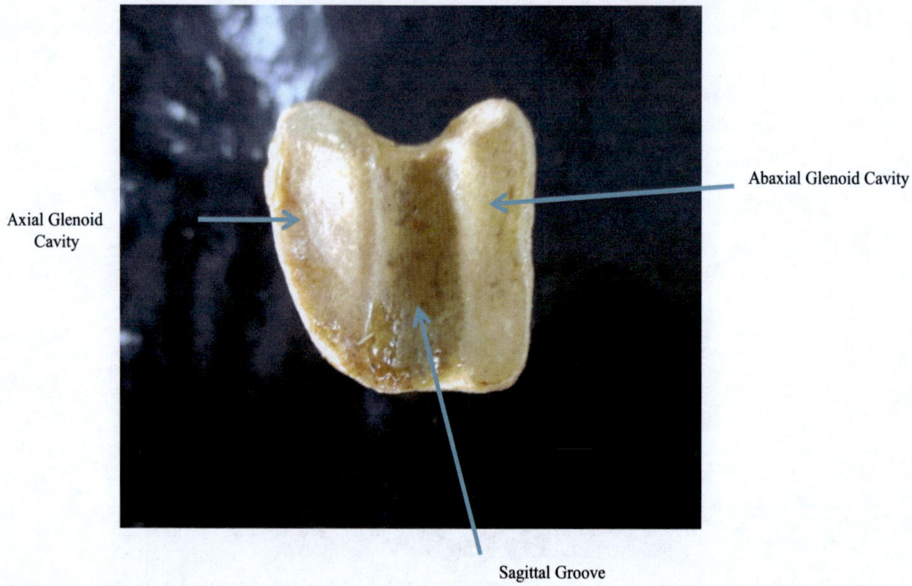

Associated Structures of Digits

1. Joints

Fetlock Joint: Between the distal metacarpals/metatarsals and the proximal phalanges.

Pastern Joint: Between the proximal and middle phalanges.

Coffin Joint: Between the middle and distal phalanges, enclosed within the hoof capsule.

2. Tendons:

Flexor Tendons (Palmar):

- **Superficial Digital Flexor (SDF)**: Inserts on P1 and P2.
- **Deep Digital Flexor (DDF)**: Inserts on P3, flexing the digit.

Extensor Tendons (Dorsal):

- **Common Digital Extensor**: Inserts on P3 of both digits.
- **Lateral Digital Extensor**: Inserts on P3 of the lateral digit.

First Phalanx (Distal Extremity)

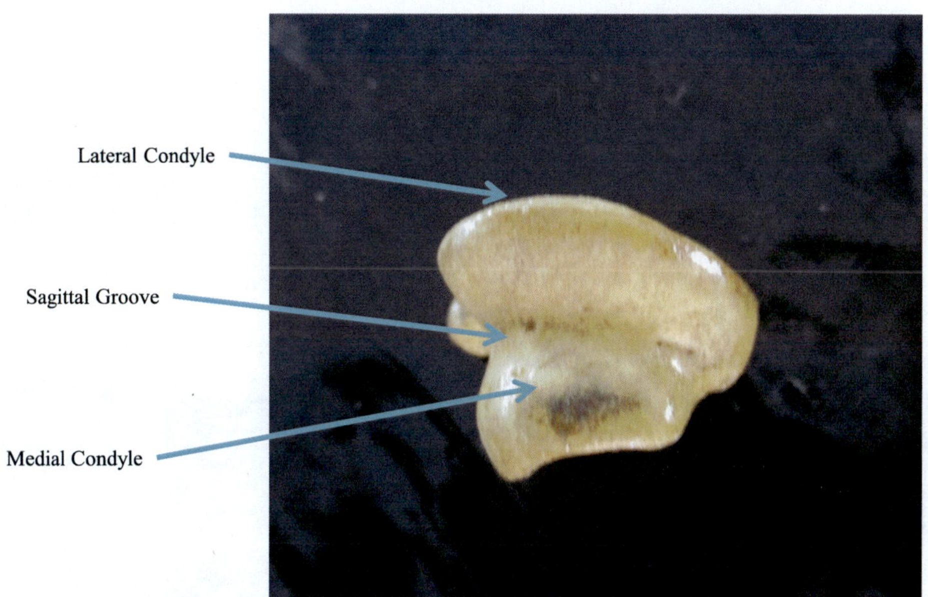

Associated Structures of Digits

3. Ligaments

Annular Ligaments: Provide stability to the tendons around the phalanges.

Collateral Ligaments: Stabilize the joints between phalanges.

4. Blood Vessels and Nerves:

- Arterial supply is primarily from the palmar digital arteries, which form loops near the coffin bone.
- Nerve supply comes from branches of the median, ulnar, and radial nerves.

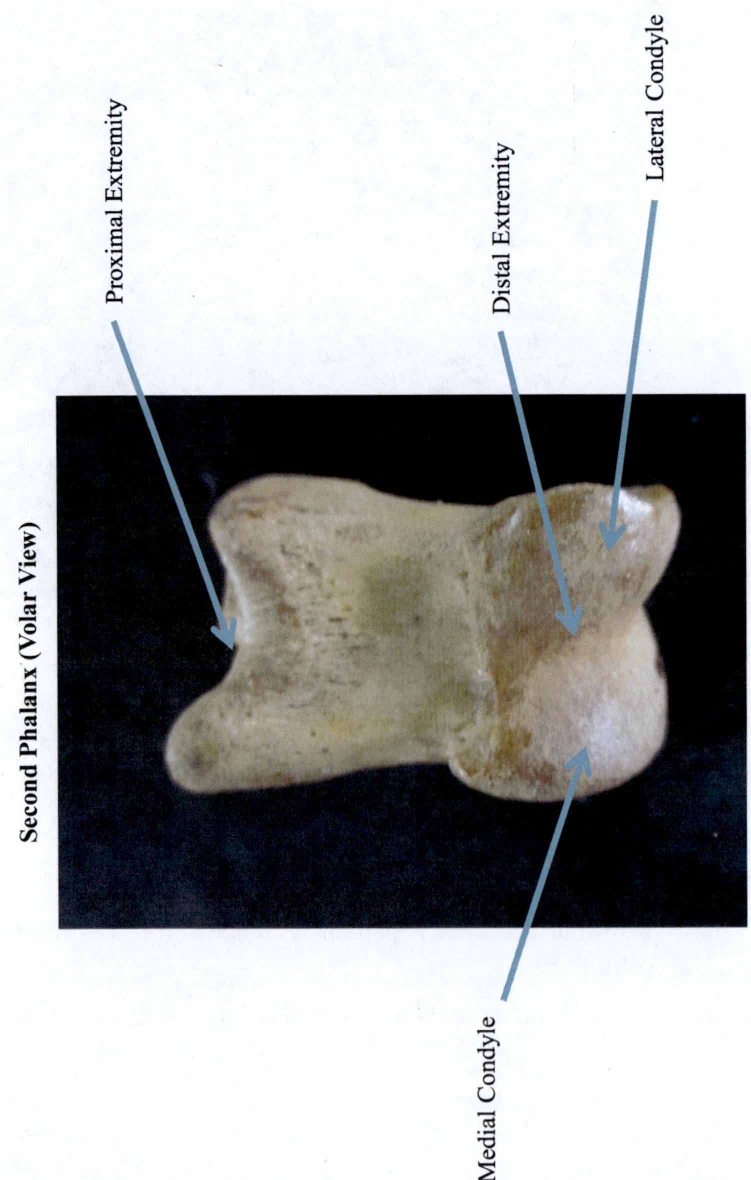

Second Phalanx (Volar View)

Clinical Significance

1. Hoof Disorders

- **Laminitis**
    - Inflammation of the laminae that attach the hoof wall to P3.
    - Causes pain, lameness, and altered weight-bearing.
- **Sole Ulcers**:
    - Develop under P3 due to pressure and poor hoof health.
    - Often associated with poor flooring or excessive standing.
- **White Line Disease**:
    - Separation of the hoof wall and sole, leading to infection and abscess formation.

2. Fractures

- **Phalangeal Fractures**
    - Common in P2 and P3 due to trauma or excessive load.
    - Signs include acute lameness, swelling, and reluctance to bear weight.
    - Treatment involves immobilization or surgical fixation.

Second Phalanx (Volar View)

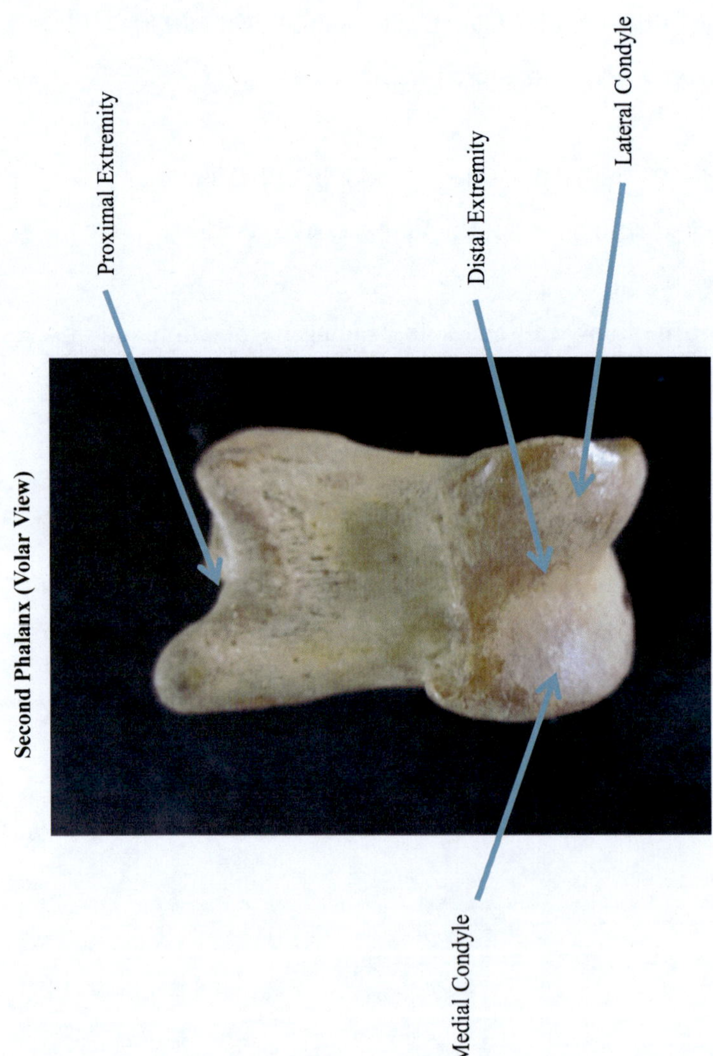

Clinical Significance

3. Joint Issues

- **Arthritis**:
  - Affects the fetlock, pastern, or coffin joints.
  - Chronic wear or infection can lead to stiffness and lameness.
- **Septic Arthritis**:
  - Resulting from penetrating wounds or systemic infections.
  - Requires aggressive treatment with antibiotics and joint lavage.

4. Tendon and Ligament Injuries

- Damage to the **flexor tendons** or **collateral ligaments** can lead to instability, abnormal gait, and pain.
- May require rest, splinting, or surgical repair.

Third Phalanx (Different Surfaces)

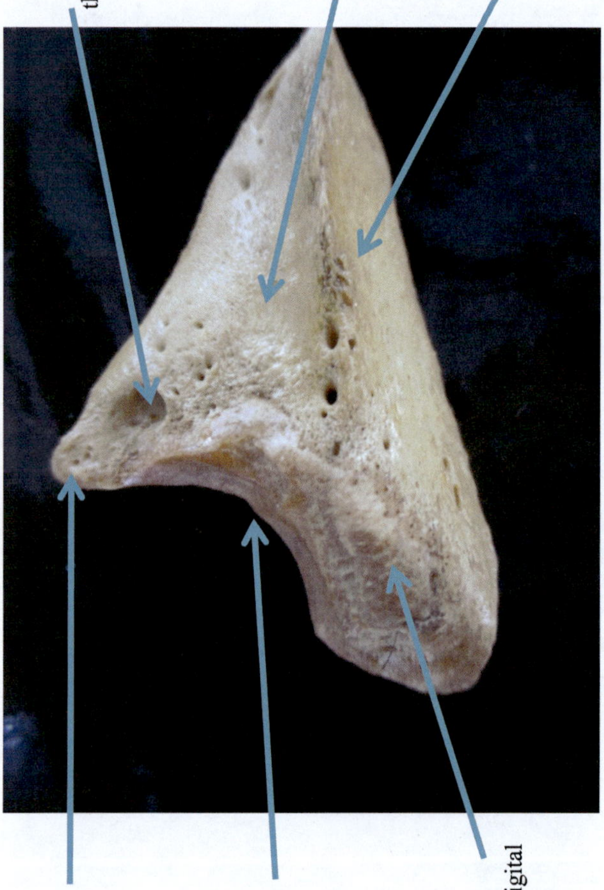

Extensor Process

Axial foramen for
the Principal artery to the hoof

Proximal Surface

Axial Surface

Tubercle
on which the deep digital
flexor attaches

Solar Surface

Clinical Significance

5. Developmental Abnormalities

- **Contracted Tendons**:
    - Congenital condition where the tendons are too short, causing the digits to curl.
    - Treated with splinting, stretching exercises, or surgical intervention.
- **Angular Limb Deformities**
    - Valgus or varus deformities can affect weight-bearing and gait.

6. Infections

- **Foot Rot**
    - Bacterial infection affecting the interdigital space, spreading to the phalanges if untreated.
    - Causes swelling, lameness, and foul odor.
- **Septic Osteitis**
    - Infection of P3 due to untreated hoof abscesses or trauma.

Bones of Hind limb

Importance of hindlimb: In cattle, the length of the hind limb is essential for effective movement, particularly during walking, trotting, or running. It influences the animal's stride length and overall agility. As quadrupeds, cattle rely heavily on their hind limbs for both weightbearing and propulsion.

Os-coxae

- Each half is made up of three bones
  a) Ilium
  b) Pubis
  c) Ischium
- Ilium
  a) Two Surfaces- Lateral and Medial
  b) Gluteal Line (on lateral surface)
  c) Ilio-Pectineal Line (divides the medial surface in to Iliac and Sacral parts)
  d) Tuber Coxae (Lateral angle)
  e) Tuber Sacrale (Medial angle)
  f) Psoas Tubercle
- Pubis
  a) Ilio-Pubic Eminence
  b) Pubic part of Pelvic Symphysis
- Ischium

a) Ischiatic Spine
b) Ischial Arch
c) Tuber Ischii
d) Greater Sciatic Notch
e) Lesser Sciatic Notch

Os-coxae (Ventral View)

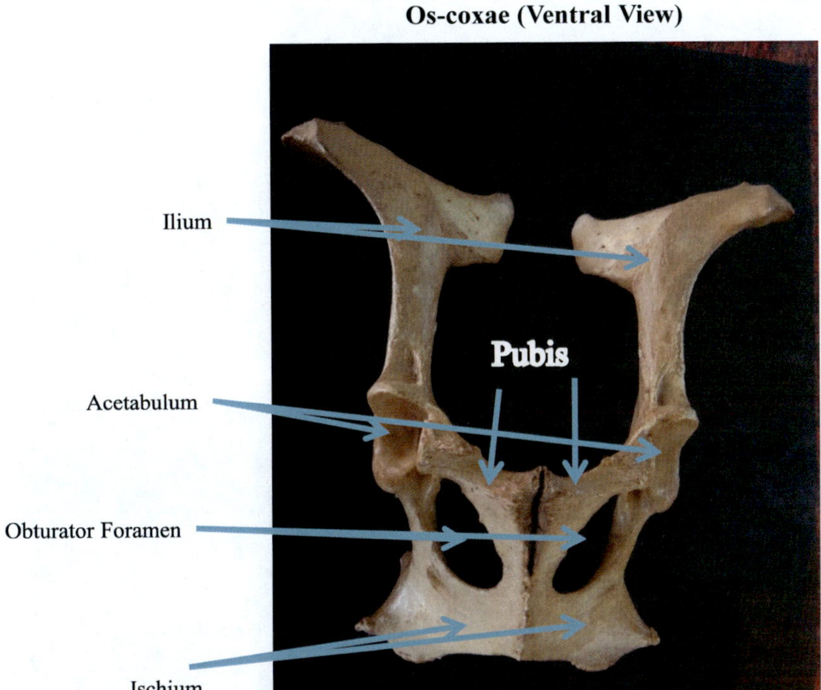

- **Pelvic brim:** The cranial edge of the pubis forms the pelvic brim and serves as the attachment point for the prepubic tendon.
- In the calf, the wing of the ilium is oriented vertically, resembling the configuration seen in dogs and other carnivores.
- However, in adult ruminants and equines, the tubera coxae are shifted laterally.

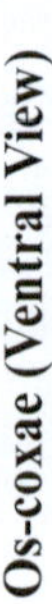

Os-coxae (Ventral View)

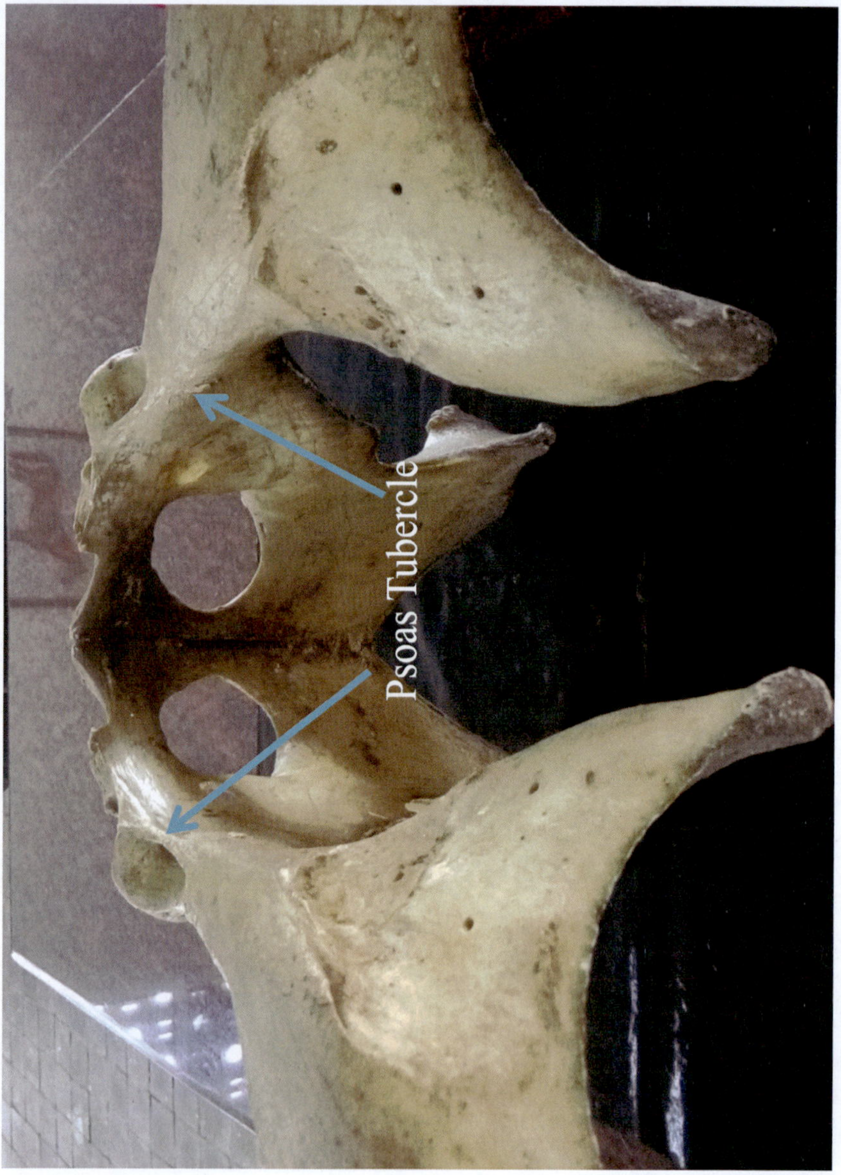

- **Pin bones:** The ischial tuberosities, commonly referred to as **'pin bones'** in cattle, form the widest part of the pelvic outlet.
- **Significance of Pin bone:** Dairy cows are evaluated and selected based on the width of their pin bones. Medially, the head of the femur articulates with the acetabulum, while the greater trochanter is located laterally, with cranial and caudal parts.
- **Birth canal:** The pelvic canal, also known as the birth canal, is the passage through which the fetus exits the female reproductive tract. The pelvic inlet and outlet define the beginning and end of this birth canal, respectively.
- **Hook bones**: In cattle, the tubera coxae are commonly referred to as "**hook bones**." A hook hoist, a clamp-like device, is often affixed to these bones to lift recumbent cattle that are unable to stand.
- The wide lateral positioning of the tubera coxae in cattle makes them particularly susceptible to fractures, especially in older animals.

Os-coxae (Dorsal View)

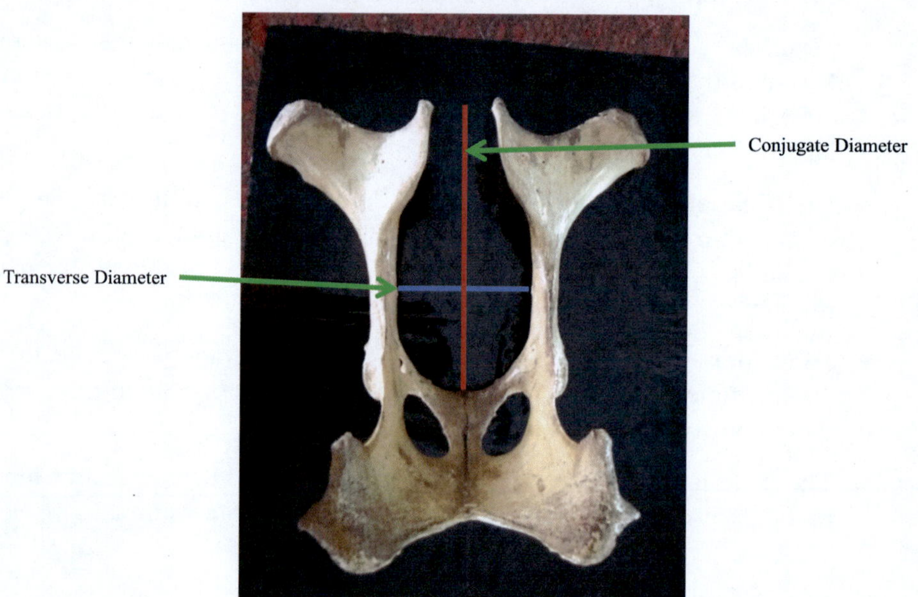

Pelvic inlet

- The pelvic inlet is the opening at the upper part of the pelvis, formed by the pelvic bones and the sacrum. It includes the wings of the sacrum, the craniomedial border of the ilium, and the pelvic brim of the pubis.
- This inlet plays a crucial role as it limits the size of the birth canal, as it is bounded by rigid bones and cannot expand. Consequently, for successful passage through the birth canal, the fetus must have a diameter smaller than that of the pelvic inlet.
- Females of various species, such as mares and cows, typically have a larger diameter pelvic inlet compared to males.
- Females of various species, such as mares and cows, typically have a larger diameter pelvic inlet compared to males.
- Consequently, for successful passage through the birth canal, the fetus must have a diameter smaller than that of the pelvic inlet.

Os-coxae (Dorsal View)

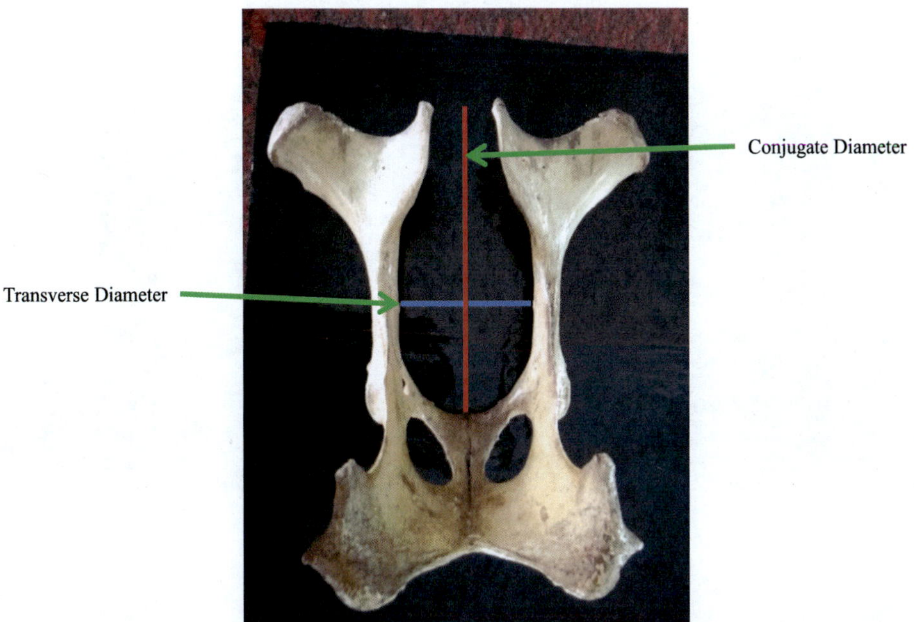

Pelvic outlet

- The pelvic outlet is the opening at the caudal end of the pelvis, formed by the caudal vertebrae, the sacrosciatic ligament (specifically its sacrotuberous part), and the ischial arch, which is the structure connecting the ischial tuberosities.
- In cattle, the ischial arch is notably deep, contributing to the unique shape of the pelvic outlet.
- This outlet is bordered by ligaments and possesses some capacity for stretching.
- The pelvic canal has two main diameters. The first, the conjugate or sacropubic diameter, is measured from the sacral promontory to the upper end of the symphysis. The second, the transverse diameter, is measured at its widest point, located just dorsal to the psoas tubercle.

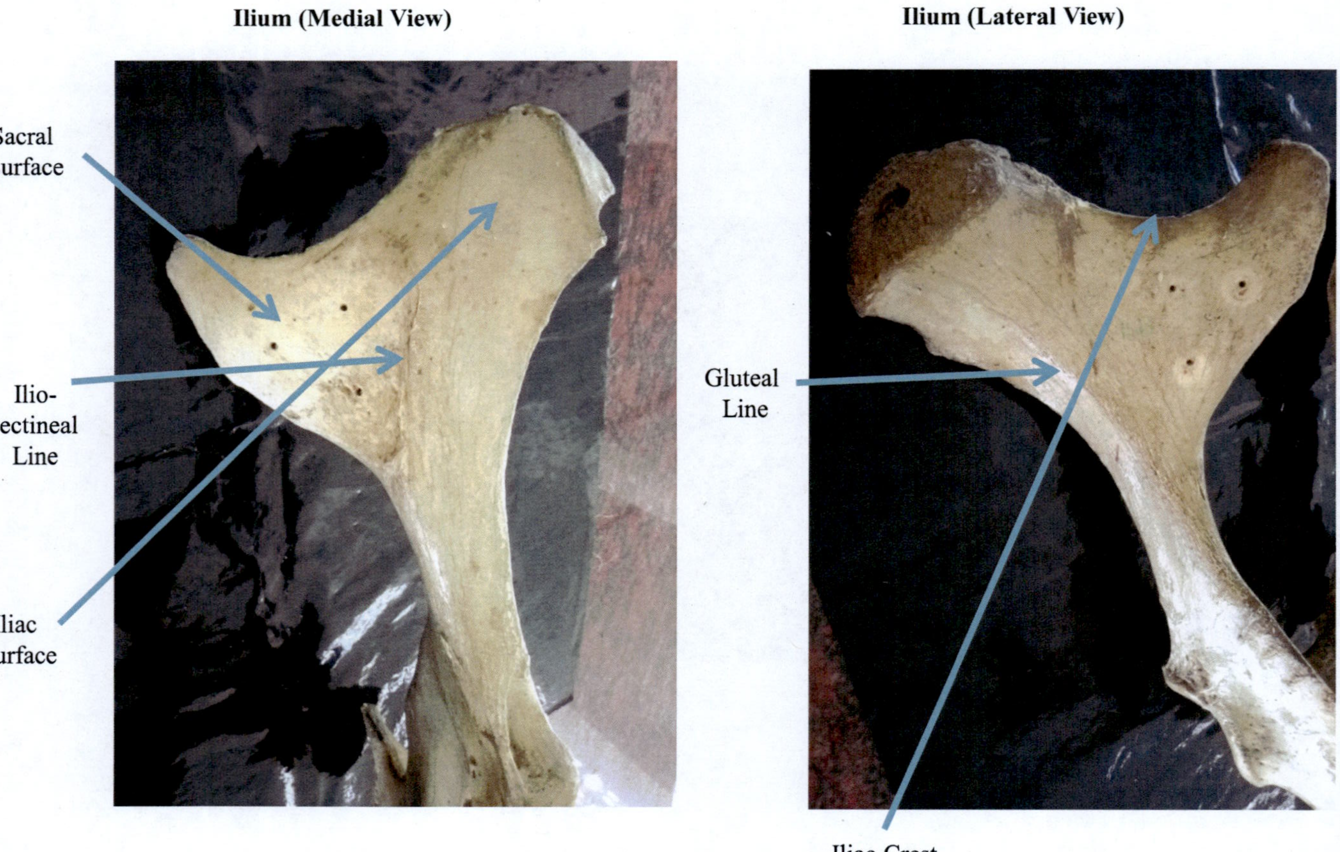
Ilium (Medial View)
Sacral Surface
Ilio-Pectineal Line
Iliac Surface
Ilium (Lateral View)
Gluteal Line
Iliac Crest

Anatomical structures related to birth canal

- During dystocia, the calf may become lodged in the birth canal, which can exert pressure on the structures within the canal.
- Several nerves originating from the lumbosacral plexus, which exit through the ventral sacral foramina, run along the inner walls of the pelvic canal.
- This pressure can lead to compression and damage to these nerves, resulting in dysfunction of the muscles they control.
- The pudendal nerve can be blocked to facilitate various procedures involving the genital and perineal areas in both males and females.

Os-coxae (Dorso-Ventral View)

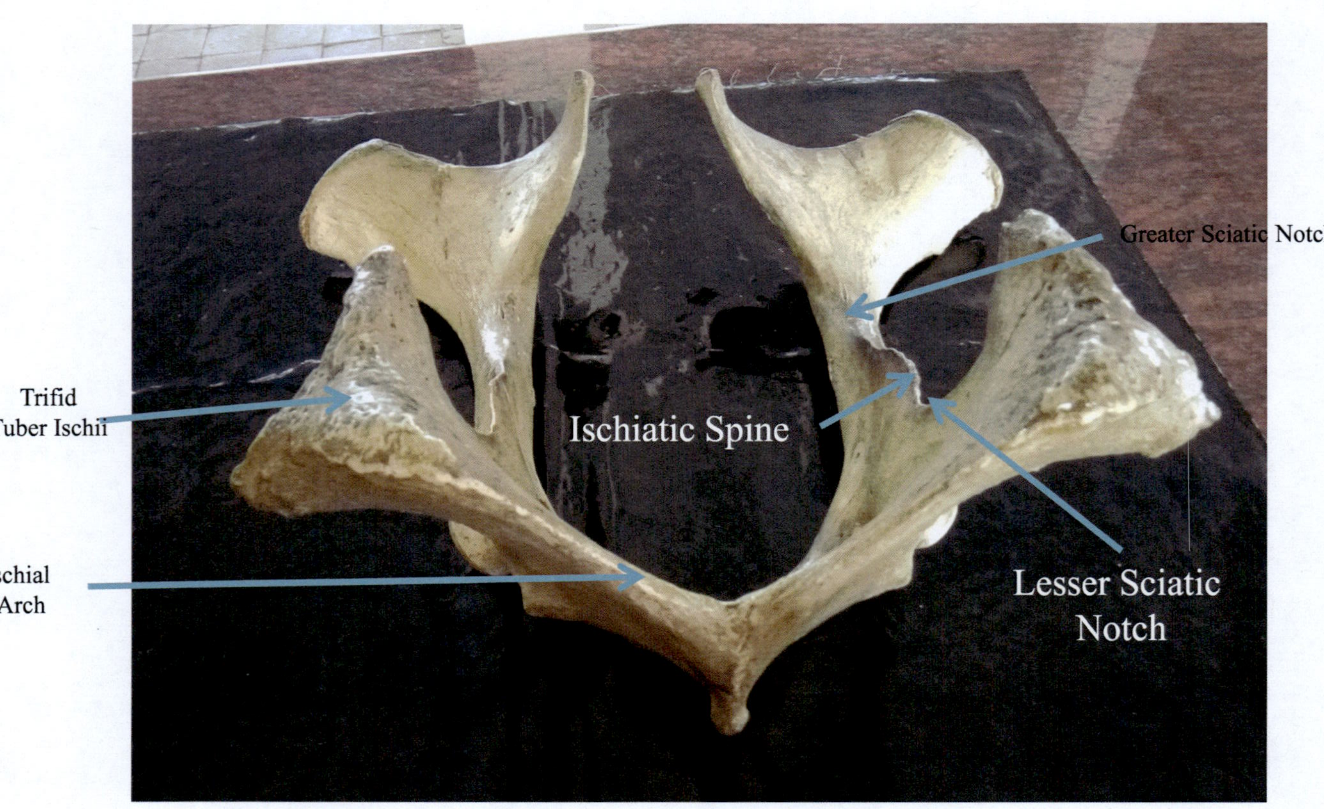

Clinical significance related to parturition of cattle

- The dimensions of the bony pelvis are important when considering dystocia.
- In calves, the pelvis's greatest width is measured across the greater trochanters, while in adult cows, it is measured across the tuber coxae.
- For successful delivery, the cow's pelvic inlet must be wide enough to allow the calf's greater trochanters to pass through.
- If the inlet is too narrow, hip lock can occur, where the calf's head and chest pass through but the greater trochanters get stuck, hindering the delivery.
- The sacrosciatic ligament, forming the upper part of the lateral wall, becomes relaxed due to hormonal changes prior to parturition. This relaxation enhances the flexibility of the sacroiliac joint, permitting the sacrum and the first few caudal vertebrae to shift dorsally. Consequently, the "high tail head" observed in preparturient cows is a result of this movement.

Femur

- **Four Surfaces**
  a) Cranial
  b) Lateral
  c) Caudal
  d) Medial
- **Proximal Extremity**
  a) Head
  b) Neck
  c) Greater Trochanter
  d) Lesser Trochanter
  e) Trochanteric Fossa
  f) Trochanteric Ridge
- **Supracondyloid Fossa**
- **Medial Supracondyloid Crest**
- **Lateral Supracondyloid Crest**
- **Distal Extremity**
  a) Cranially Trochlea
  b) Caudally Condyles
  c) Extensor Fossa
  d) Intercondyloid Fossa

Femur (Caudal View)

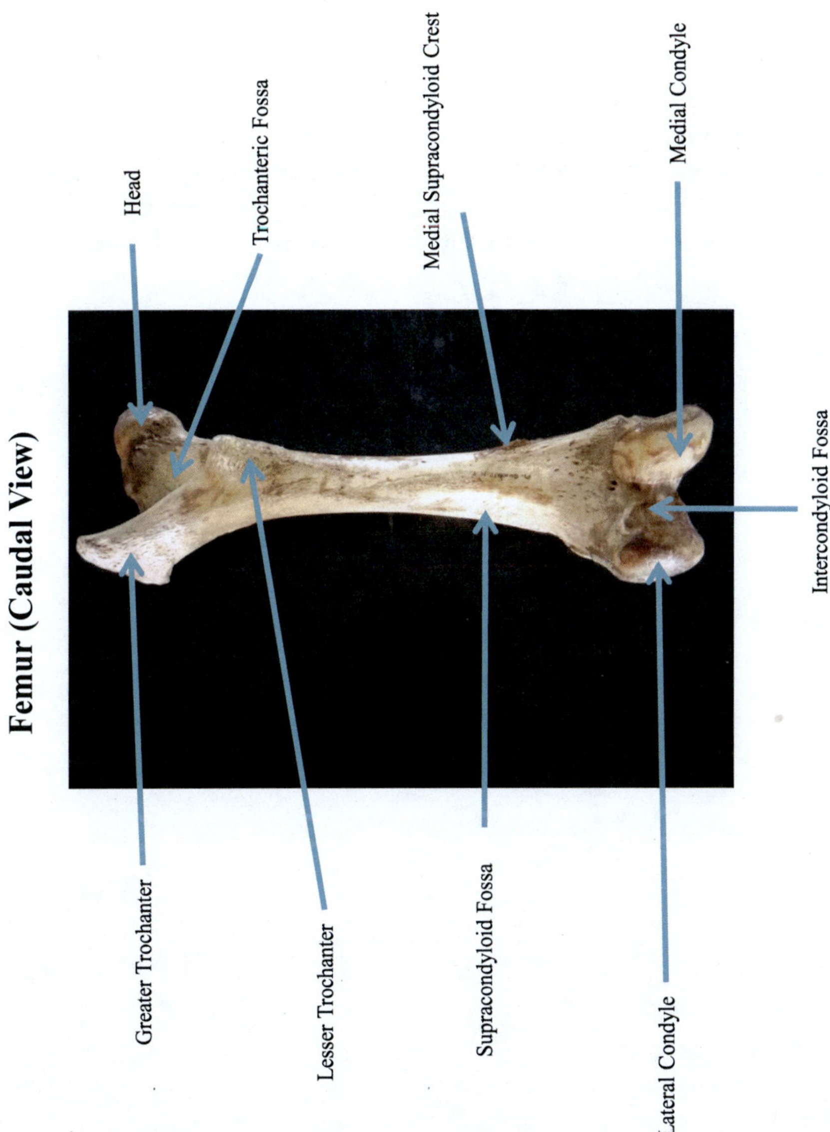

- **The sciatic nerve** exits near the greater sciatic foramen, which is formed by the sacrosciatic ligament.
- It then travels caudally around the hip joint, medial to the greater trochanter, and continues distally in the pelvic limb.
- In **downed animals**, particularly cows, the nerve can become compressed against the caudal surface of the upper femur.
- **Pelvic diaphragm:** The coccygeus and levator ani muscles originate from the pelvic bones and insert onto the caudal vertebrae of the tail and the region around the anus. Together, they form the pelvic diaphragm, which plays a crucial role in supporting the rectum and other pelvic organs, helping to prevent herniation. These muscles are particularly significant in small animals, such as dogs, where weakness in this area is commonly linked to the development of perineal hernias.

Femur (Proximal Extremity)

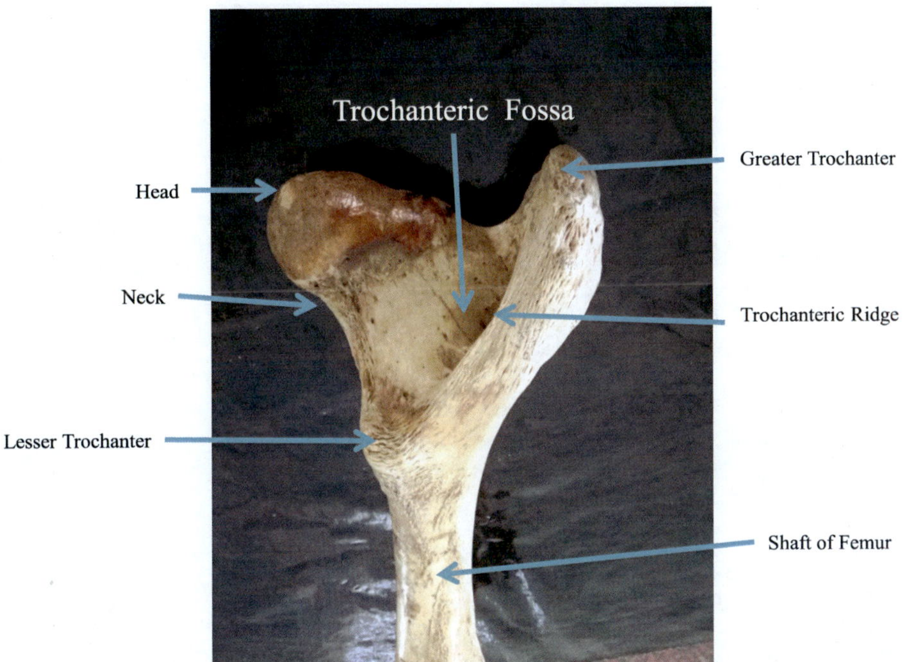

Hip joint dislocation

- Dislocation refers to a condition where the normal contact between articulating bones is completely lost. This is also referred to as luxation in some cases, while a partial loss of contact is termed subluxation.
- Hip joint dislocation can result from major trauma or can occur as a secondary complication of hip dysplasia.
- Hip dysplasia is a congenital condition that typically affects both sides, characterized by a misalignment between the femoral head and the acetabulum. A common feature of hip dysplasia is an abnormally shallow acetabulum, which causes joint instability and can lead to degenerative joint disease (DJD). Although hip dysplasia is most frequently observed in large dog breeds, it can also occur in other domestic animals such as cattle.

Femur (Proximal Extremity)

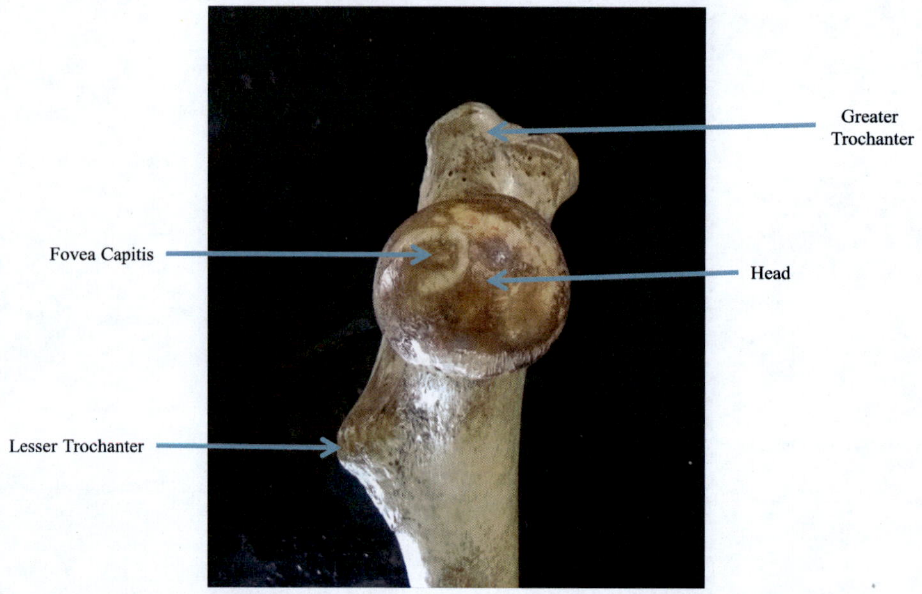

Proximal part of Femur

- The femur, commonly known as the thigh bone, is the heaviest bone in the body.
- The head of the femur contains a centrally located fovea, which serves as the attachment site for the round ligament of the femoral head.
- The greater trochanter is undivided and located laterally on the femur.
- The middle gluteal muscle is one of the most powerful extensors of the hip joint. This is due to its attachment to the lever provided by the greater trochanter. It plays a crucial role in propelling the pelvic limb caudally during actions like kicking and also assists the animal in rearing up on its hind limbs.
- The sciatic nerve travels caudally around the hip joint, passing medially to the greater trochanter, and extends distally along the pelvic limb.
- In recumbent animals, especially cows, the sciatic nerve may become compressed against the caudal surface of the upper femur.

Femur (Lateral View)

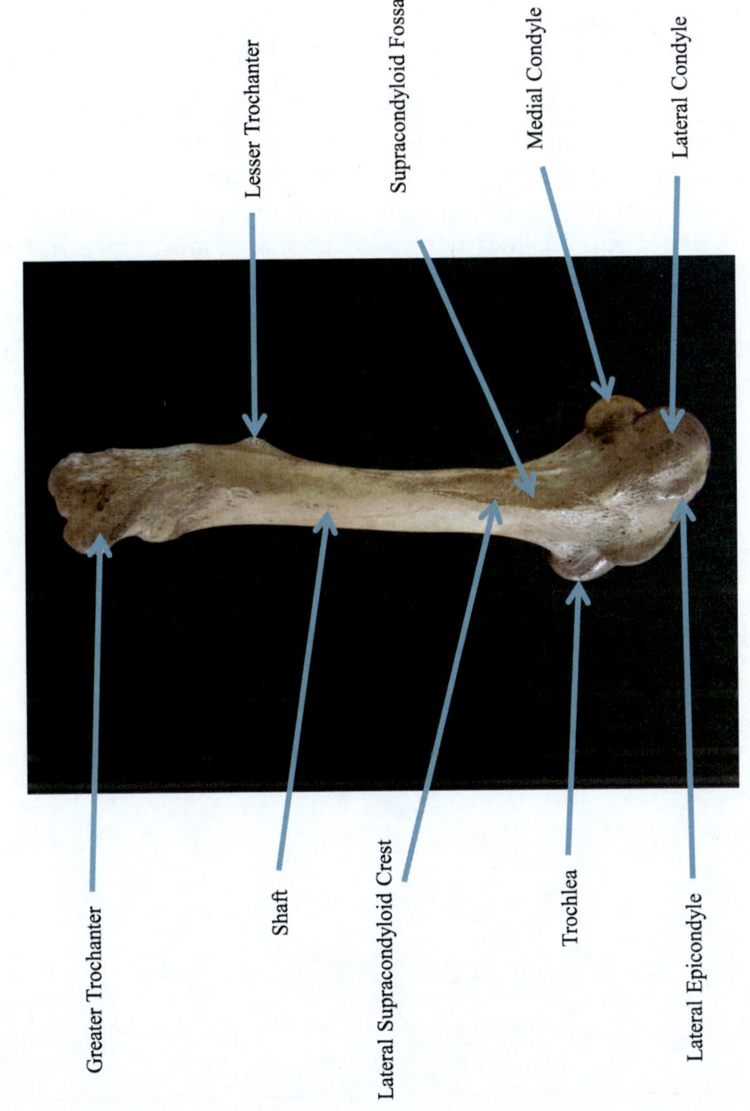

Distal part of Femur

- The trochlea is located on the cranial surface of the distal end of the femur, with the medial ridge being larger than the lateral ridge.
- The quadriceps femoris is the primary muscle responsible for extending the stifle joint and is innervated by the femoral nerve. If the femoral nerve is damaged or anesthetized, the limb loses its ability to support weight.
- The saphenous nerve, a branch of the femoral nerve, travels distally alongside the saphenous artery on the medial surface of the limb within the **femoral triangle**. The femoral artery, femoral vein, and saphenous nerve pass between the two origins of the sartorius muscle on their way to the femoral triangle. The sartorius forms the medial wall of the triangle, with the pelvic tendon of the external oblique creating the proximal border, the gracilis and pectineus muscles forming the caudal border, and the rectus femoris forming the cranial border.

Femur (Medial View)

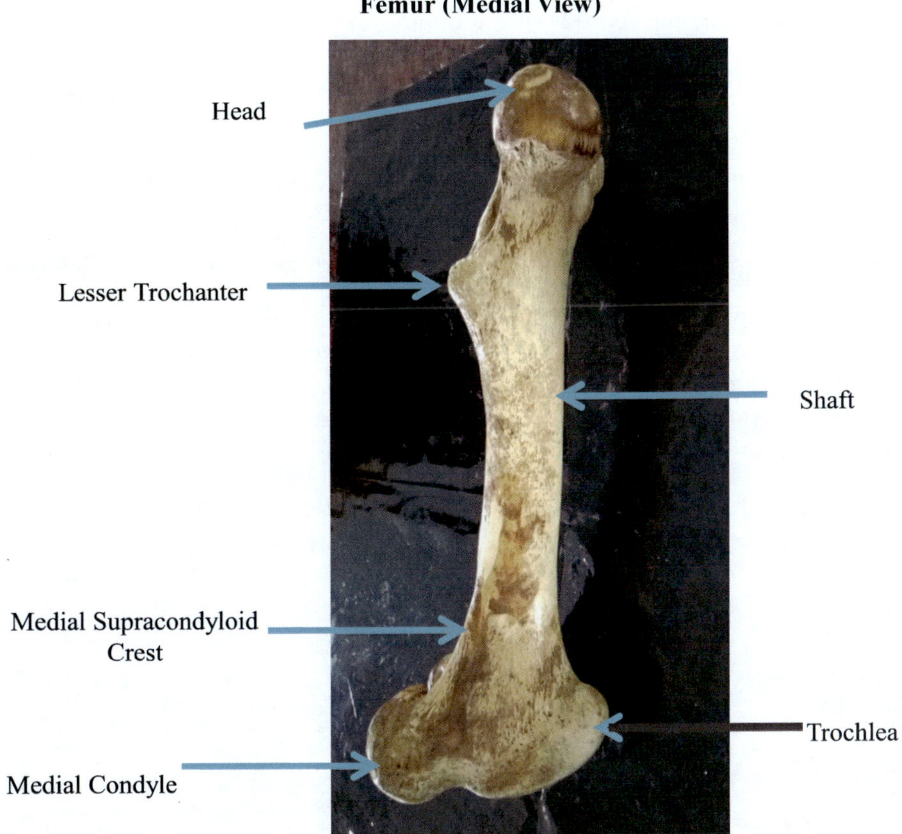

Distal part of Femur

- At the distal end of the femur, the femoral trochlea features a prominent medial ridge and a smaller lateral ridge. This area is a common site for osteochondrosis, a condition where cartilage separates from the underlying bone, leading to joint lesions.
- The distal femur features medial and lateral condyles that articulate with the meniscal cartilages.
- Located between these condyles is the intercondylar fossa, which serves as the attachment site for the cranial and caudal cruciate ligaments.
- On the distal portion of the lateral femoral condyle there is extensor fossa, the origin point for the long digital extensor and fibularis (peroneus) tertius muscles.
- Additionally, the supracondylar fossa is situated on the caudolateral aspect of the femur, just proximal to the lateral condyle. This fossa is where the superficial digital flexor muscle originates.

Femur (Distal Extremity)

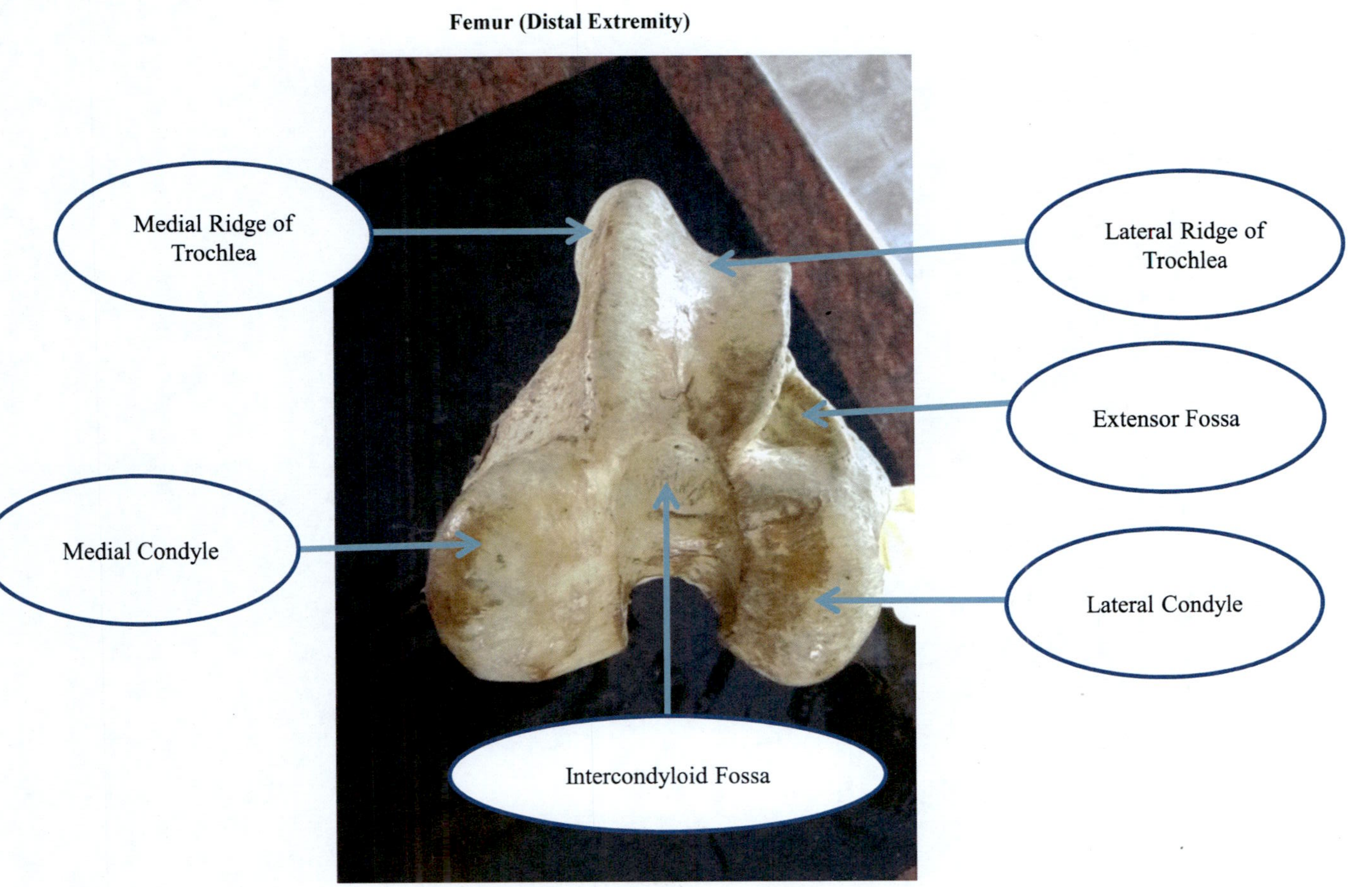

Hamstring muscle

- The hamstring muscle group consists of the biceps femoris, semitendinosus, and semimembranosus muscles. In ruminants, the superficial gluteal muscle is fused with the biceps femoris, forming a single muscle known as the gluteobiceps.
- These hamstring muscles play a key role in shaping the pelvic (croup) region. In cattle, the pelvis tends to appear more angular or sunken, which is due to the structure of their hamstring muscles. Specifically, ruminants possess only pelvic heads—portions of the muscles that originate from the ischiatic tuberosity and extend downward. They lack vertebral heads, meaning no part of the muscle arises from the caudal vertebrae to overlay the hip bone.
- In contrast, horses have hamstring muscles with both vertebral and pelvic heads, giving their croup a more rounded and muscular appearance.

Clinical condition related to hip and thigh joints

Joint	Feature	Clinical
Sacroiliac joint	Creates a strong connection between the hind limb and the trunk.	Dislocation possible
Hip joint	Deep socket; accessory ligament (equine)	Bovine – Luxation can occur; Equine – Luxation is unlikely due to two strong ligaments securing the femoral head in the socket.
Stifle joint	Both equines and bovines have three patellar ligaments and three joint compartments with variable interconnections. In equines, a patellar locking mechanism is present	Patellar fixation

Patella

- **Two Surfaces**

    a Free

    b Articular

    - Apex
    - Base
    - Two Borders

    a Lateral

    b Medial

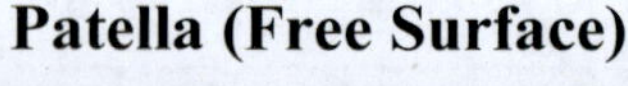

Patella (Free Surface)

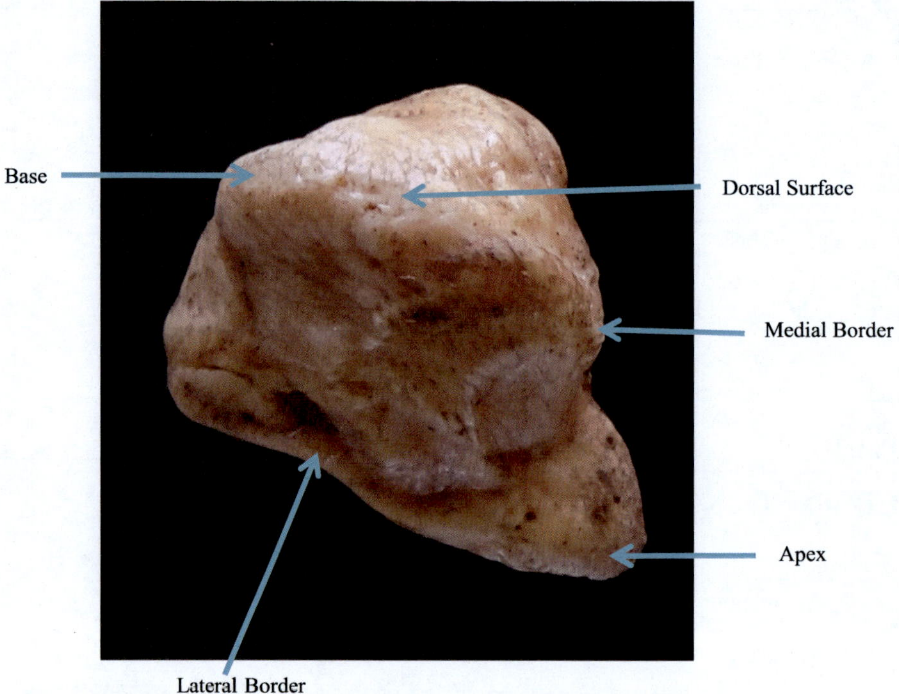

The patella

- The patella is the largest sesamoid bone that gradually develops within a tendon and articulates trochlea of femur.
- Its broad base is oriented proximally and has a roughened surface for muscle attachment, while the pointed apex faces distally.
- Functionally, the patella redirects the pull of the quadriceps femoris muscle, absorbs pressure, and transmits force through the patellar ligament to the tibial tuberosity. The patellar ligament is essentially a continuation of the quadriceps femoris tendon.

Patella (Articular Surface)

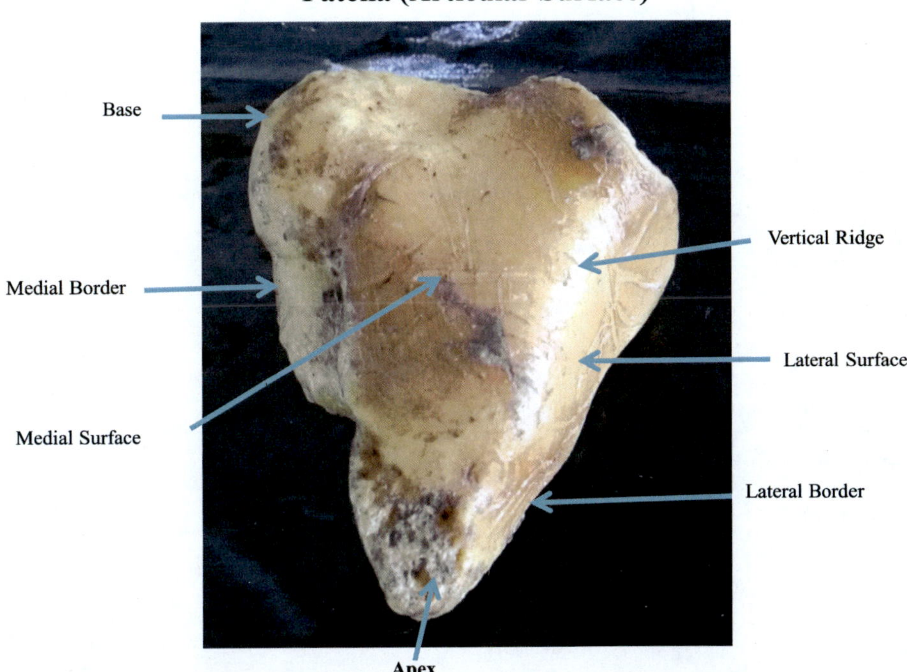

Upward fixation of the patella

- In horses and ox, the patella is anchored to the tibial tuberosity by three separate ligaments: the medial, intermediate, and lateral patellar ligaments, named according to their position.
- A clinical condition known as **upward fixation of the patella** (or patellar fixation) can occur in some cattle breeds. This disorder prevents the stifle joint from unlocking, resulting in a stiff-legged gait. To correct this, a surgical procedure called medial patellar desmotomy may be performed, in which the medial patellar ligament is severed near its attachment to the tibial tuberosity.
- Additionally, a structure known as the patellar fibrocartilage connects the medial patellar ligament to the patella, reinforcing this attachment.

Tibia

- **Three Surfaces**

  a) Lateral

  b) Caudal

  c) Medial

- **Proximal Extremity**

  a) Medial Condyle

  b) Lateral Condyle

  c) Spine

  d) Sulcus Muscularis

  e) Intercondyloid Fossa

  f) Popliteal Notch

  g) Tibial Crest

  h) Tibial Tuberosity

- **Distal Extremity**

  a) Facets for Lateral Malleolus

  b) Medial Malleolus

  c) Sagittal Facets for Tibial Tarsal

  d) Articular Groove

  - **Popliteal Line (on Caudal surface)**

  - **Tubercle for Cruciate Ligament (on Caudal surface near proximal extremity)**

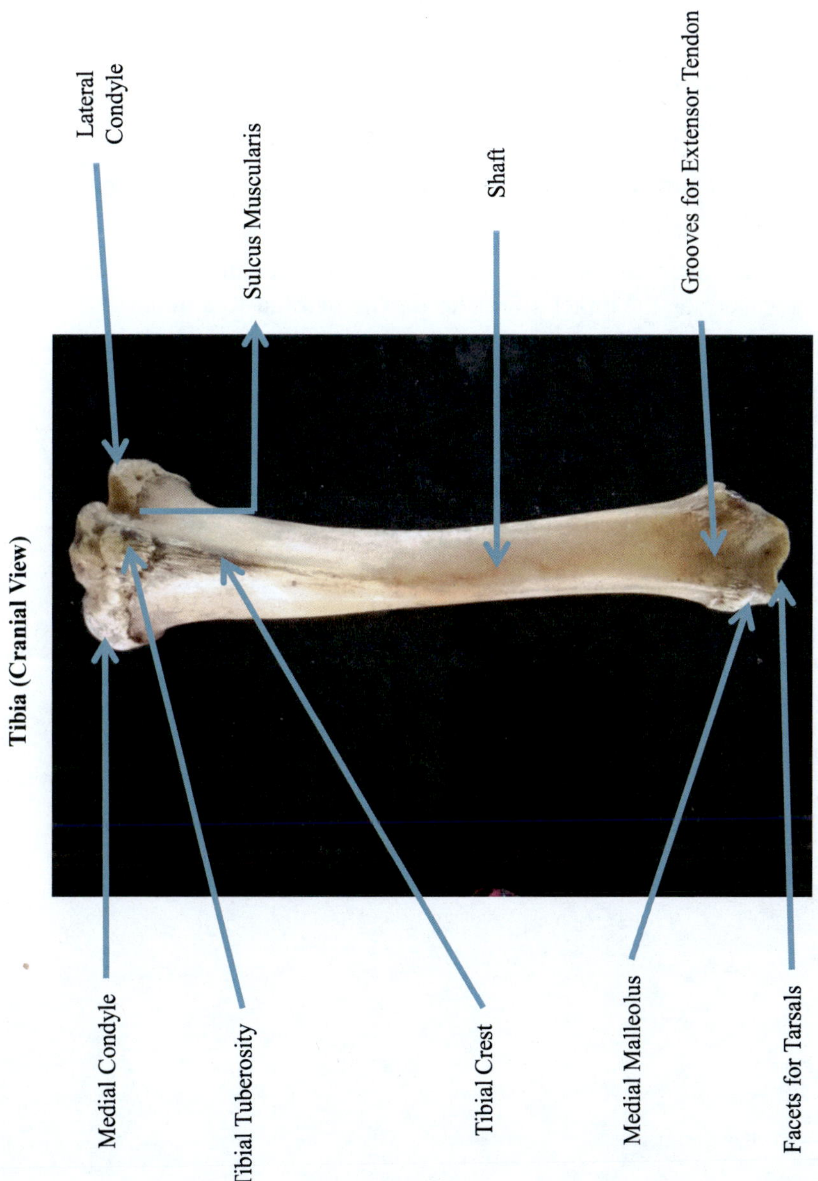
Tibia (Cranial View)
Lateral Condyle
Sulcus Muscularis
Shaft
Grooves for Extensor Tendon
Medial Condyle
Tibial Tuberosity
Tibial Crest
Medial Malleolus
Facets for Tarsals

- **The leg skeleton** is composed of the tibia and fibula. The tibia is a long bone located medially. The fibula lies lateral to the tibia.
- The proximal end of the tibia features the medial and lateral condyles.
- These tibial condyles articulate with the condyles of the femur, aided by fibrocartilaginous discs known as the menisci.
- Between the tibial condyles lies the intercondylar eminence.
- The medial surface of the tibia is largely subcutaneous, making it easily palpable.
- **The tibial tuberosity**, found on the proximal and anterior surface of the tibia, serves as the attachment site for the patellar ligament.

Tibia (Caudal Surface)

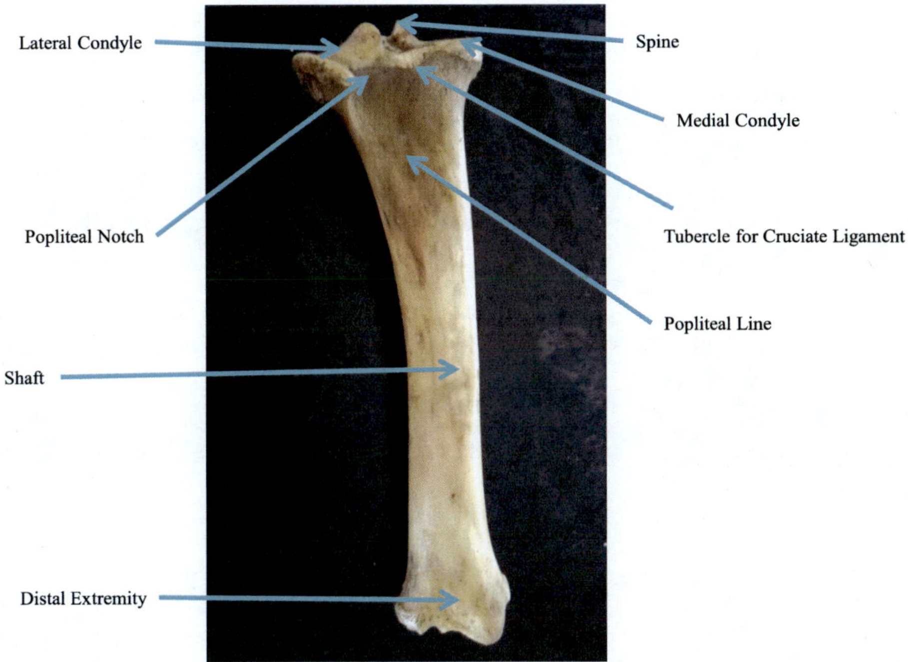

Proximal part of Tibia

- **The sulcus muscularis** (also known as the **extensor groove**) separates the tibial tuberosity from the lateral condyle and serves as a passageway for the tendons of the extensor muscles.
- The tibia, with its medial and laterally projecting lateral condyles, presents proximal articular surfaces that lie nearly at the same level.
- Cranial and caudal to the intercondyloid eminence are the intercondyloid fossae, which serve as attachment sites for the cranial cruciate ligament and the menisci.
- The condyles are separated caudally by the deep popliteal notch, and on its medial side is a tubercle for the attachment of the caudal cruciate ligament.

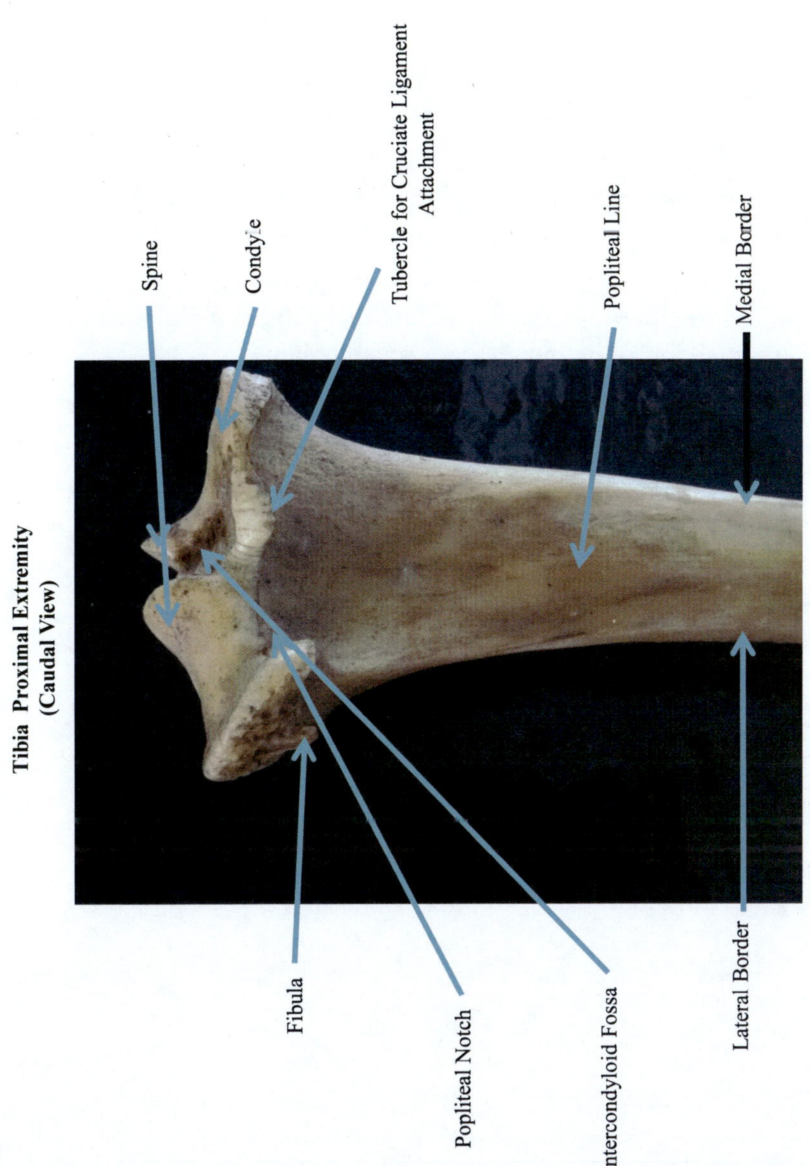
Tibia Proximal Extremity
(Caudal View)
Spine
Condyle
Tubercle for Cruciate Ligament Attachment
Popliteal Line
Medial Border
Fibula
Popliteal Notch
Intercondyloid Fossa
Lateral Border

Distal part of Tibia and Fibula

- The distal extremity bears the cochlea, which articulates with the tibial tarsal. The articular ridge and grooves of the cochlea are oriented almost in the sagittal plane.
- On the lateral surface of the cochlea, there are two articular facets for articulation with the distal segment of the fibula, known as the lateral malleolus.
- The proximal portion of the fibula is fused to the lateral condyle of the tibia, forming a process that is directed distally.
- In ruminants, most of the fibular shaft is undeveloped and typically replaced by a fibrous strand, resulting in the distal end of the fibula—the lateral malleolus—remaining as a separate bone.
- The lateral malleolus articulates proximally with the tibia, medially with the talus, and distally with the calcaneus. The fused medial malleolus forms a process that is directed distally.

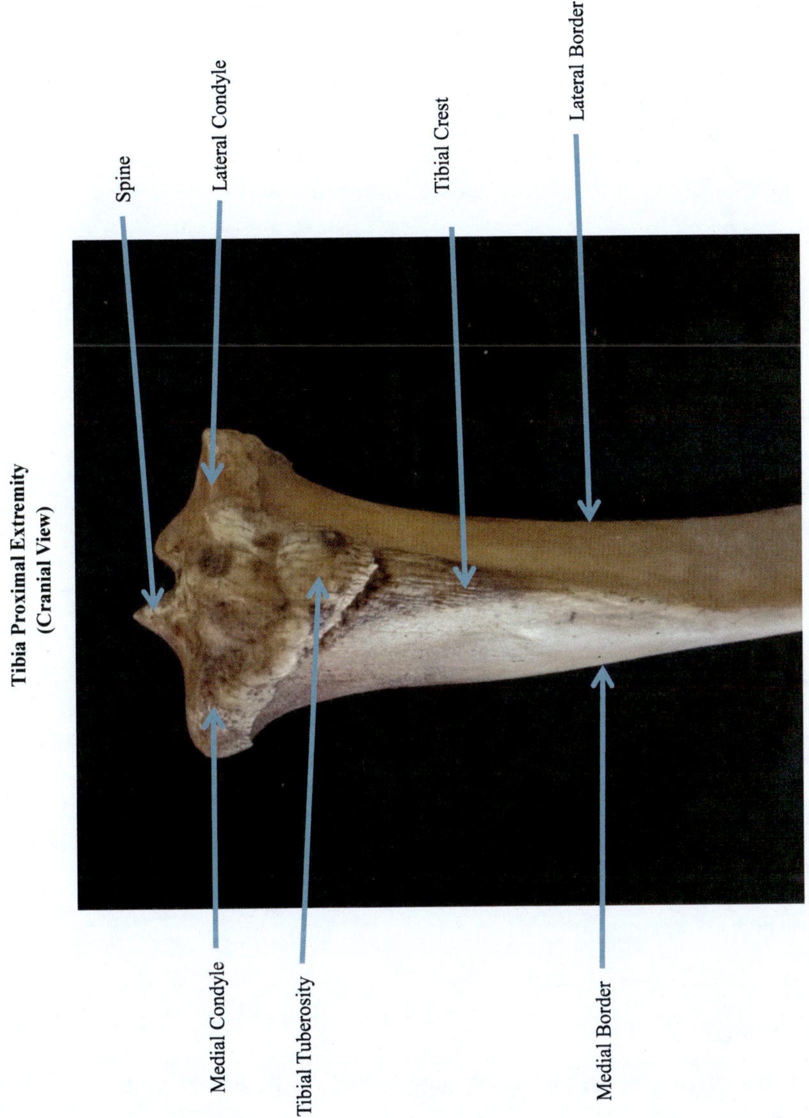

**Tibia Proximal Extremity
(Cranial View)**

Clinical conditions related to bovine leg

Rupture of the anterior cruciate ligament (ACL)

- Increased laxity in the stifle joint
- Audible clicking or popping during joint movement
- Joint effusion present

Medial collateral ligament (MCL) rupture

- Widened medial joint space
- Medial meniscal instability

Peroneus Tertius Rupture

- Overextension of the hock
- Tibia and metatarsus can extend to 180°
- Swelling present on the cranial aspect of the tibia

Peroneal Neuropathy

- Overextended hock
- Knuckling of the fetlock
- Decreased skin sensation on the dorsal surface of the metatarsus and fetlock

Tibial Neuropathy

- Dropped hock
- Knuckling of the fetlock
- Loss of skin sensation on the palmar aspect of the lower limb

Tibia (Proximal Extremity)

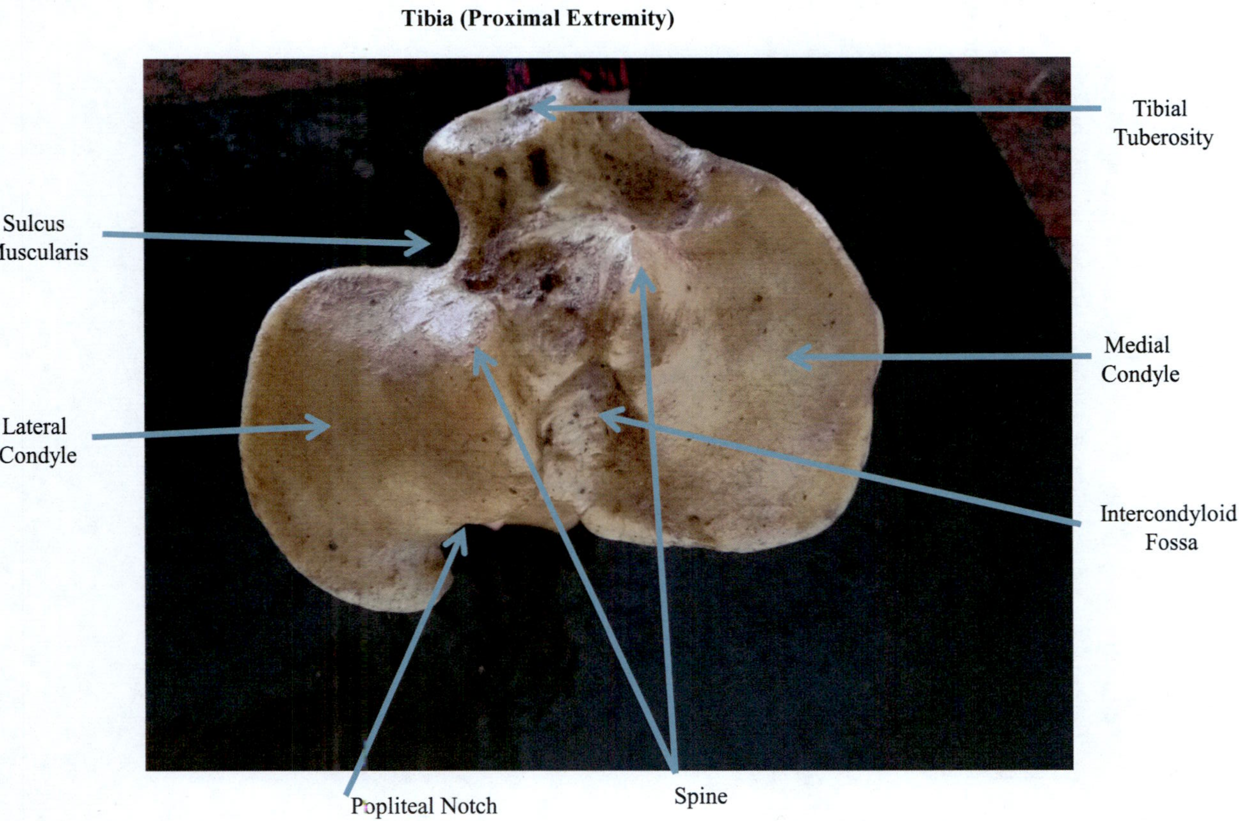

Tibial or peroneal nerve paralysis

- Tibial or peroneal nerve paralysis commonly occurs in cattle following parturition or after prolonged recumbency, primarily due to pressure-induced ischemia over the lateral aspect of the stifle.
- Affected animals typically present with hyperflexed fetlocks, and in some cases, may walk on the dorsum of the fetlock. Although they are able to bear weight on the limb, the hock appears overextended, and the animal is unable to extend the digits. When associated with prolonged labor, both hindlimbs are often affected. This condition is considered a milder form of sciatic nerve injury.
- Treatment involves bandaging or splinting to help realign and support the fetlock. Differential diagnoses include gastrocnemius rupture, which typically presents with a more pronounced drop in the hock. Recovery generally takes 2 to 3 months.

Tibia (Distal Extremity)

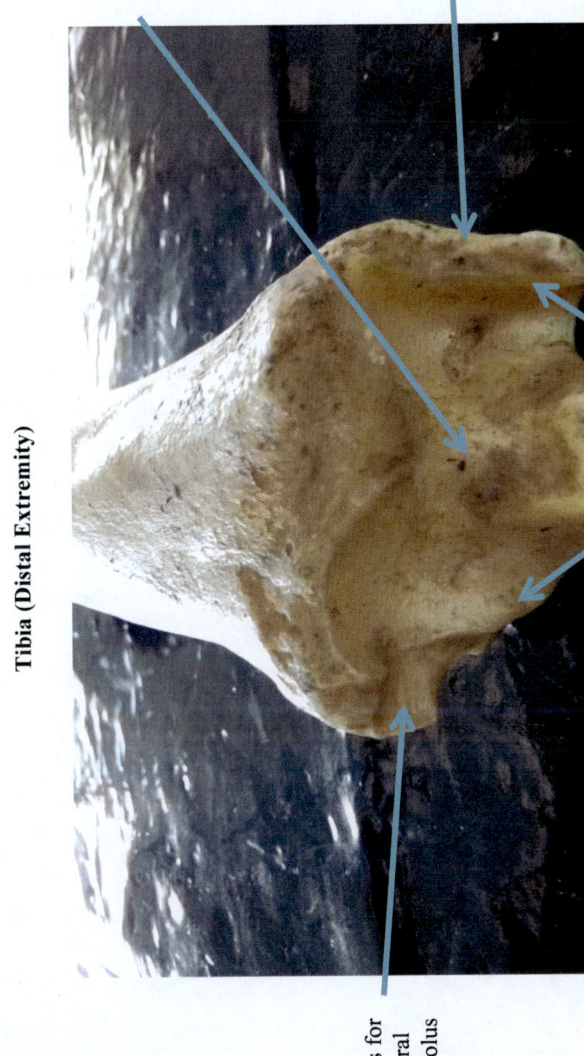

Joint trauma and sepsis in leg

- Arthrocentesis is a valuable diagnostic tool for distinguishing between joint trauma and sepsis. In nonseptic cases, the total cell count in synovial fluid typically remains below 1,000 cells/mL, with polymorphonuclear cells comprising less than 10% of the total.
- When performing arthrocentesis of the stifle, it's important to understand the joint anatomy. The femoropatellar and medial femorotibial joint compartments usually communicate, but this connection doesn't always extend to the lateral femorotibial compartment.
- To access the lateral compartment, insert the needle behind the lateral patellar ligament and direct it caudally. For the femoropatellar and medial femorotibial compartments, insert the needle between the medial and middle patellar ligaments, angling it slightly downward and medially toward the medial lip of the trochlea

Damage of medial collateral ligament

- When the medial collateral ligament is damaged, the medial meniscus can become detached, and the joint capsule may stretch, leading to increased looseness on the medial side of the joint.
- The affected limb is typically held in an abducted position, placing more weight on the medial claw. If the leg is pulled outward, the joint space on the medial side becomes noticeably wider, which can be felt by palpation.
- Additionally, the medial meniscus may show excessive movement, which can be detected by palpating the area between the medial collateral ligament and the medial patellar ligament..

Tarsals

- **Bones are arranged in three rows**
  - a) Proximal
  - b) Middle
  - c) Distal
- **Proximal Row**
  - a) Tibial
  - b) Fibular
  - c) Middle Row
  - d) Fused Central and Fourth
- **Distal Row**
  - a) First
  - b) Second and Third Fused

Tarsal Bones (Lateral View)

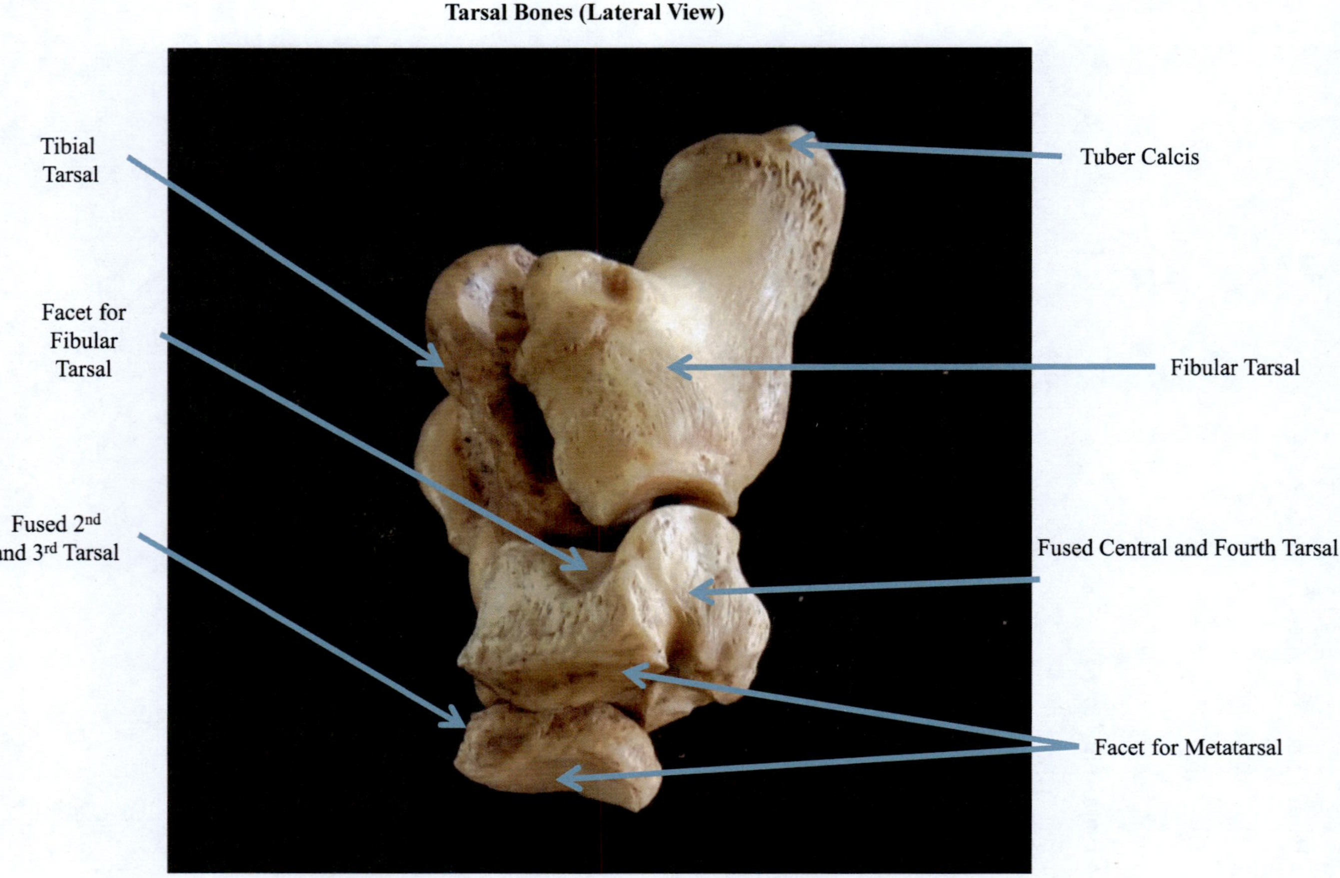

Rupture of the peroneus muscle

- Rupture of the peroneus muscle leads to overextension of the hock joint, as this muscle group primarily functions to flex the joint. In cattle, such ruptures commonly occur either in the muscle belly or at the junctions where the tendon meets the muscle proximally or distally.
- When the affected limb is manually lifted and extended backward, the tibia and metatarsus align in a straight line, while the stifle joint remains bent at a 90-degree angle.
- This injury typically causes noticeable pain and swelling over the front (cranial) aspect of the tibial shaft.

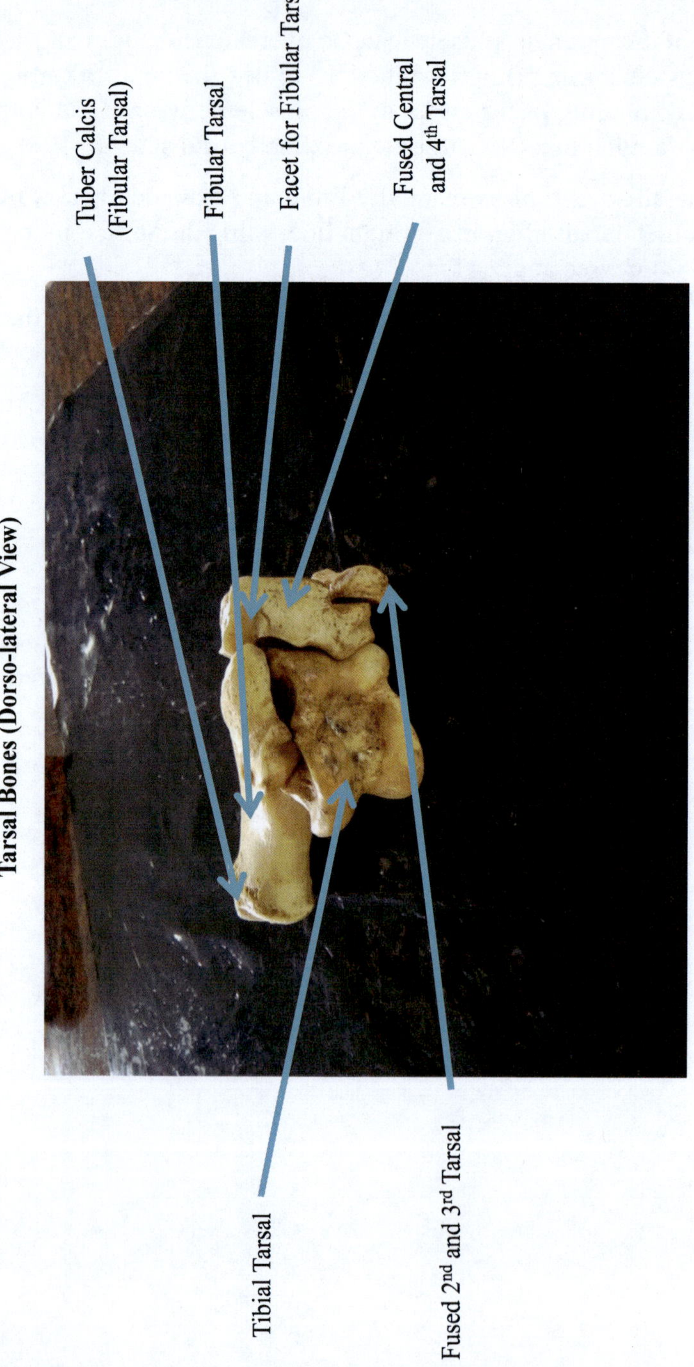

Tarsal Bones (Dorso-lateral View)

Peroneal neuropathy in cow

- Peroneal neuropathy in cow can lead to loss of sensation on the dorsal side of the lower limb and cause overextension of the leg.
- The peroneal nerve runs superficially along the lateral rear leg, making it susceptible to injury, especially in cows with milk fever or downer cow syndrome. In these cases, prolonged pressure from the cow's body weight can damage the nerve as it crosses over bone. Affected cows often show an overextended hock joint.
- In mild cases, the fetlock may occasionally knuckle over during walking, while in more severe cases, sensation around the dorsal fetlock is reduced. Recovery varies based on the severity of the injury, ranging from a few days to several months.

Tibial Tarsal (Dorsal view)

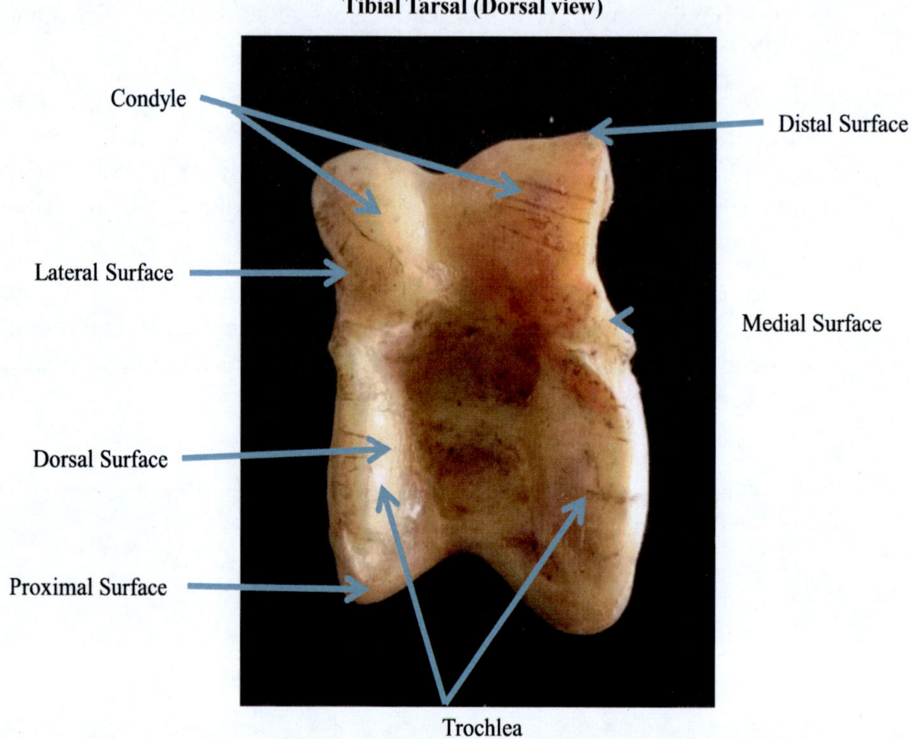

- **The talus** in bovine features two trochleae: a proximal trochlea, which corresponds to the single trochlea found in the horse, and a distal trochlea.
- On the **calcaneus**, notable landmarks include the calcanean tuberosity, which projects caudally and laterally, and the sustentaculum tali, located medially.
- **Clinical Note:** In ruminants and camelids, the presence of two trochleae allows for increased tarsal flexion, providing a greater range of motion compared to species with only one trochlea.

Tibial Tarsal (Plantar view)

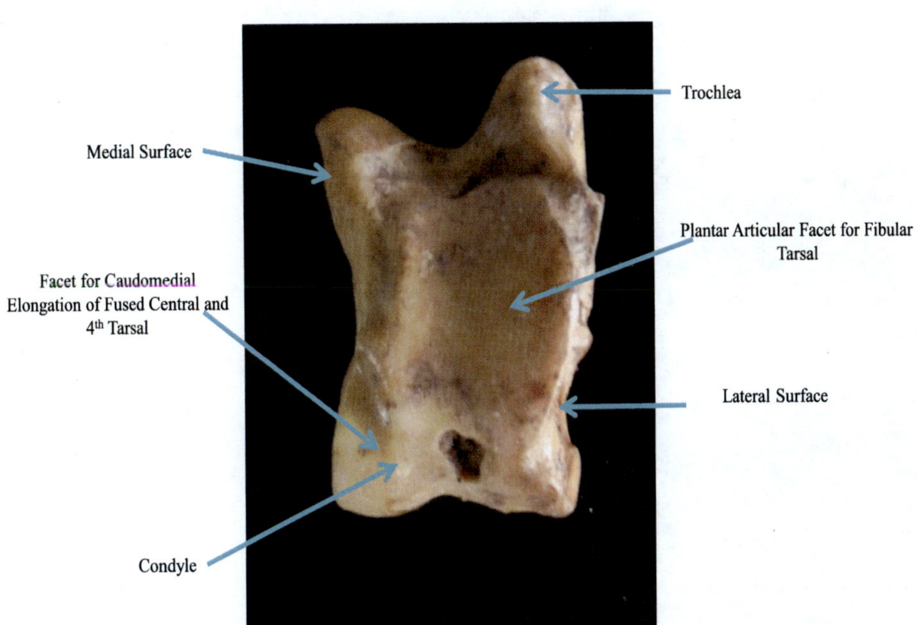

Gastrocnemius muscle rupture

- Overflexion of the hock is a characteristic sign of gastrocnemius muscle rupture. Swelling is typically present at the site of injury. The gastrocnemius muscle originates from the caudal surface of the femur and inserts on the point of the hock, specifically the tuber calcanei.
- Rupture can occur in three locations: within the muscle belly, at the muscle–tendon junction (the most common site), or at the tendon's insertion on the tuber calcis. Diagnosis is based on classic clinical signs, including overflexion of the hock, tendon laxity, and localized swelling or edema.
- Differential diagnoses include calcanean bursitis, luxation of the superficial digital flexor tendon, and tarsal fractures. In cases of complete rupture, the animal is typically recumbent and unable to rise. A key diagnostic indicator of complete rupture is the ability of the animal to fold the affected limb entirely onto itself.

Tibial Tarsal (Medial View)

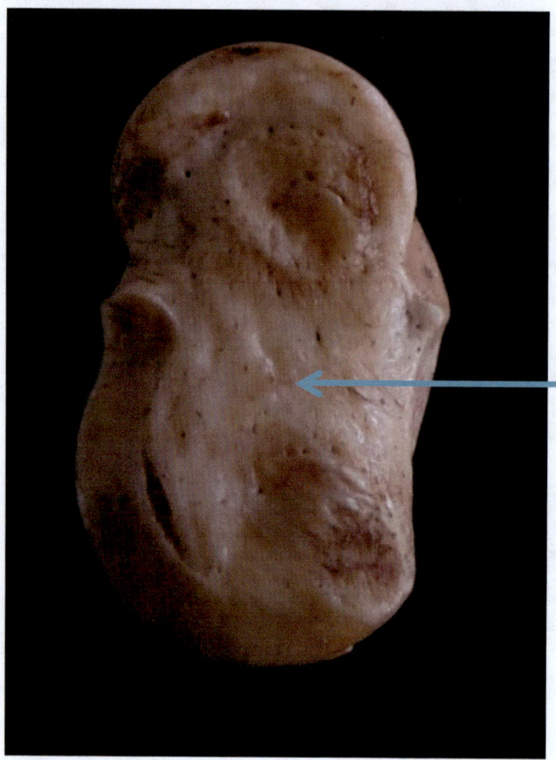

Swelling of the hock joint

- Swelling of the hock joint is commonly linked to peritarsal bursitis, septic arthritis, or degenerative joint disease, which may occur with or without post-legged conformation.
- Peritarsal bursitis is a chronic inflammation (cellulitis) affecting the lateral side of the hock, and it typically presents on both hind limbs.
- Lameness is generally not observed unless the swelling interferes with joint movement or is complicated by severe abscess formation or septic arthritis. In such advanced cases, the animal may become markedly lame, often with a draining tract on the lateral side of the hock.
- The affected area may feel warm, soft (fluctuant), and painful when touched or moved. A needle aspirate can confirm the presence of exudate, aiding in diagnosis.

Tibial Tarsal (Lateral View)

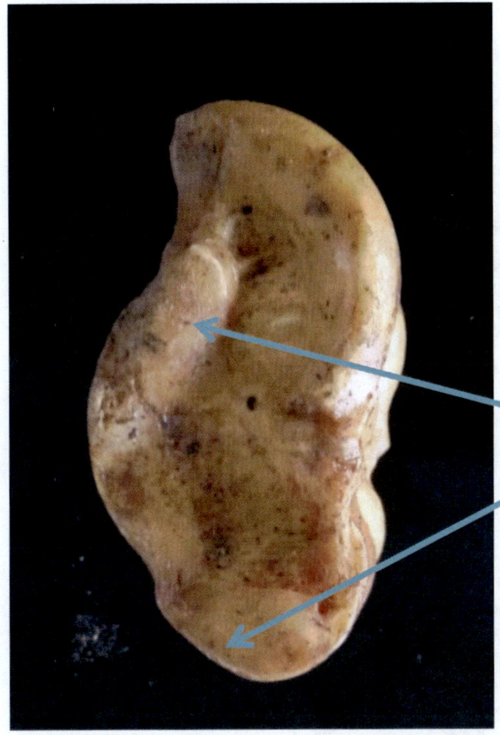

Articular Surfaces on the Lateral Surface for the Fibular Tarsal

Tibial neuropathy

- The tibial nerve supplies sensation to the plantar (underside) surface of the hind limb. In cases of tibial neuropathy, this can result in partial or complete loss of sensation.
- Partial injury to the sciatic nerve—often caused by calving or spinal trauma—is typically bilateral. Affected cows exhibit short, stilted steps, with both hocks and fetlocks held in semiflexion.
- A thorough spinal palpation and rectal examination are recommended to check for possible fractures.

Fibular Tarsal (Medial View)

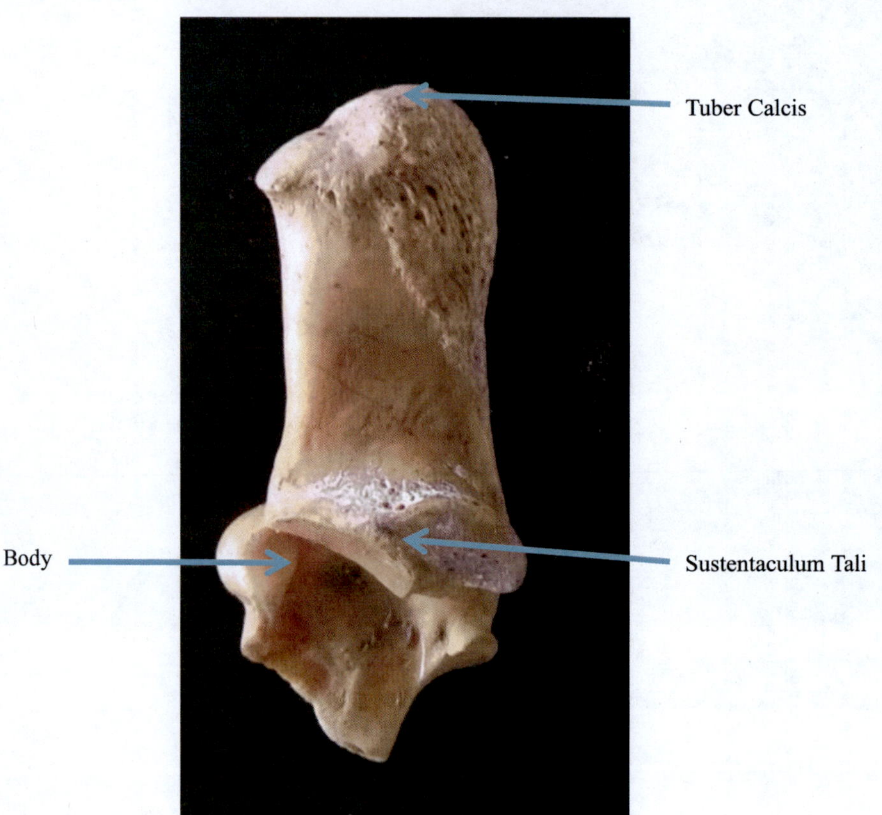

Peritarsal abscess

- A peritarsal abscess must be differentiated from a septic joint, and ultrasound is a useful tool for this distinction.
- The tibiotarsal pouch communicates with the proximal intertarsal compartment but does not extend into the distal intertarsal or tarsometatarsal compartments.
- On ultrasound, a peritarsal abscess appears as a walled-off fluid-filled cavity located outside the joint, often showing a cellular or complex internal appearance.

Fibular Tarsal (Lateral View)

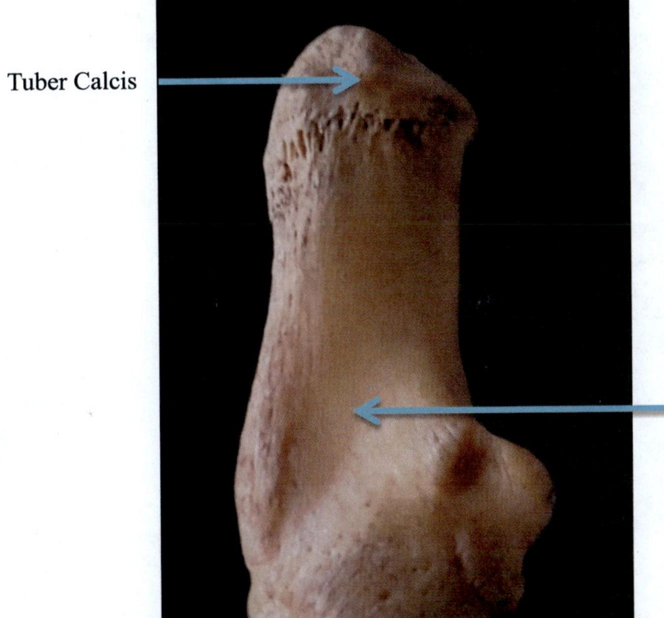

Chronic degenerative joint disease

- In cases of chronic degenerative joint disease, joint swelling tends to be firm and less painful compared to the more acute inflammation seen with septic tarsitis. For diagnostic or therapeutic procedures, the needle is inserted on the dorsal aspect of the joint, just medial to the extensor tendons and at the level where the tibia articulates with the proximal tarsal bones.
- Degenerative changes in the joint may also be linked to chronic infections, including those caused by Mycoplasma species. These chronic bone alterations can often be visualized through radiographic imaging.

Fibular Tarsal (Distal Extremity)

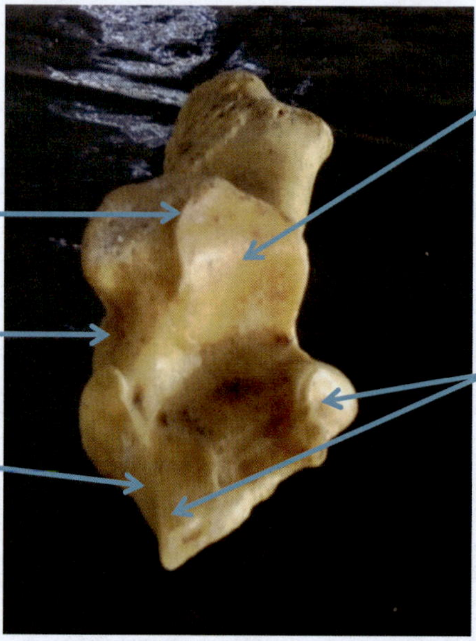

Facet for Plantar Surface of Tibial Tarsal

Sustentaculum Tali

Body

Facets for Lateral Surface of Tibial Tarsal

Facet for Fused Central and Fourth Tarsal

Quadriceps Femoris Muscle

- The quadriceps femoris is the largest muscle located on the cranial surface of the femur. It is composed of four distinct heads: the rectus femoris, vastus lateralis, vastus medialis, and vastus intermedius. The three vastii muscles—vastus lateralis, vastus medialis, and vastus intermedius—originate from the proximal region of the femur. In contrast, the rectus femoris arises from the ilium, specifically from a site cranial to the acetabulum.
- Distally, all four heads of the quadriceps femoris converge to form a common tendon, which inserts onto the tibial tuberosity via three patellar ligaments. Functionally, the quadriceps femoris serves as a principal and powerful extensor of the stifle (knee) joint. Among its four heads, the rectus femoris is unique in that it also crosses the hip joint, contributing to flexion of the hip.

Fused Central and 4th Tarsal (Proximal View)

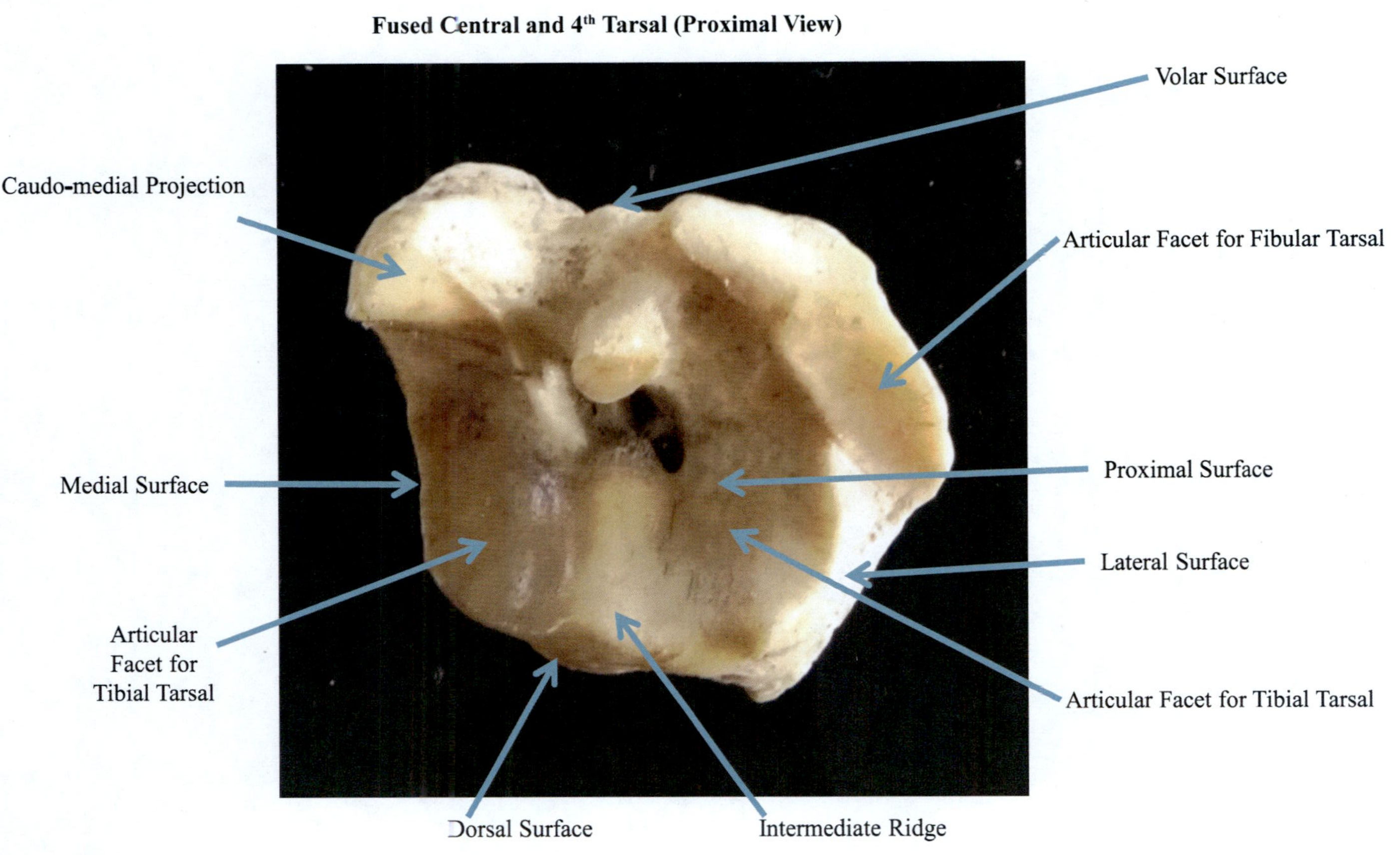

Peroneal nerve paralysis (additional points)

- Peroneal nerve paralysis is a common secondary complication associated with conditions such as milk fever, downer cow syndrome, or any situation where a cow remains recumbent for an extended period. In more severe cases, affected cows may show reduced sensation on the dorsal surface of the fetlock.
- Overextension of the fetlock can also occur as a result of flexor tendon rupture or damage to the suspensory ligaments of the proximal sesamoid bones. This overextension may become so pronounced that the animal bears weight on the plantar or palmar surface of the foot. Swelling may be observed just above the dewclaws, and ultrasound examination may reveal effusion within the tendon sheath or core lesions in the flexor tendons.

Fused Central and 4th (Distal View)

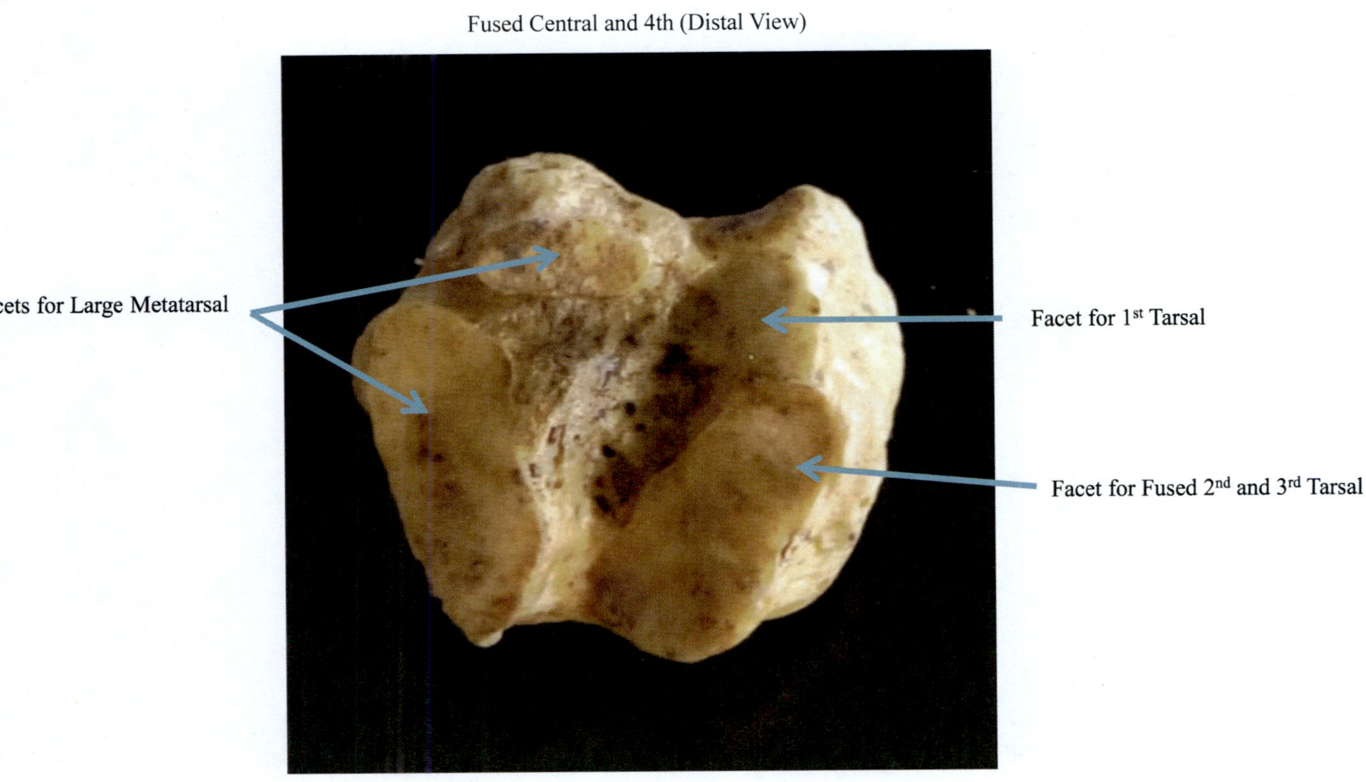

Muscles Acting on the Hock and Digits

- The muscles of the crus are divided into two main groups based on their position and function:

Craniolateral Group: This group includes muscles that either:

- Flex the hock only, or
- Flex the hock and extend the digits. These muscles are innervated by the common peroneal (fibular) nerve, a branch of the sciatic nerve.

Caudomedial Group: This group consists of muscles that either:

- Extend the hock only, or
- Extend the hock and flex the digits. These muscles are innervated by the tibial nerve.

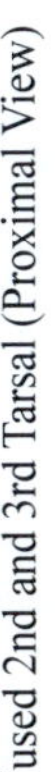

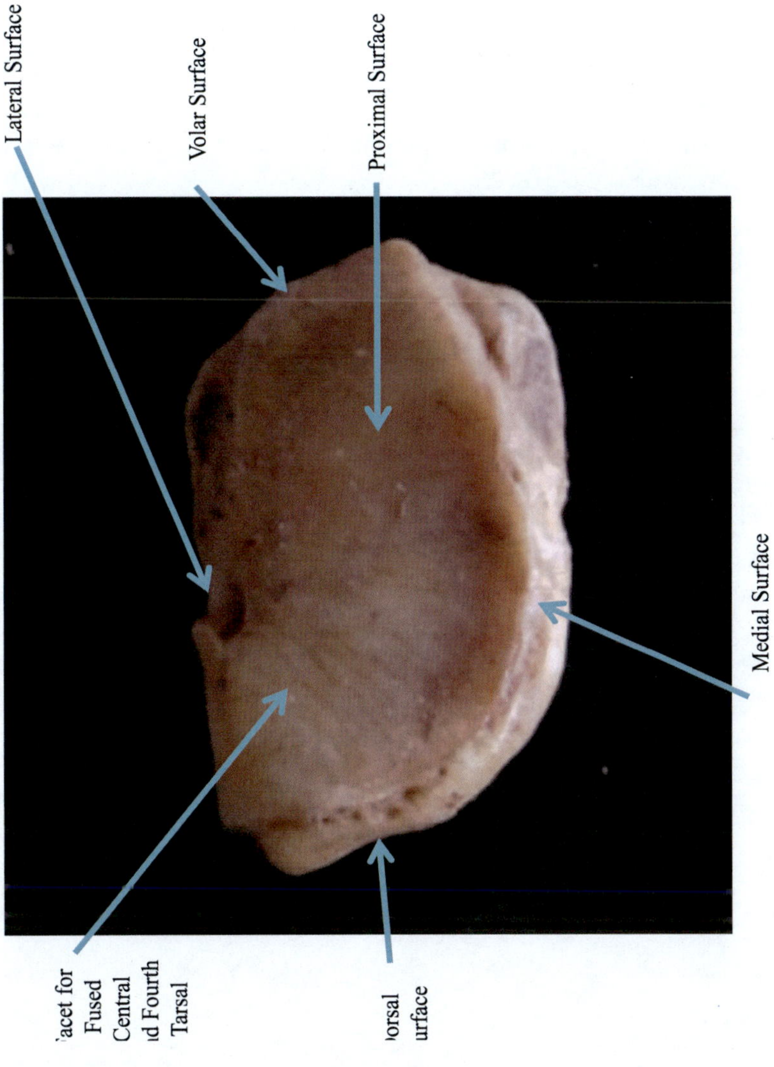

Fused 2nd and 3rd Tarsal (Proximal View)

Craniolateral Muscles of the Leg (Crus)

- The craniolateral group of leg muscles includes the cranial tibial fibularis (peroneus) tertius, long digital extensor, short digital extensor, fibularis (peroneus) longus, and lateral digital extensor muscles.
- The terms fibularis and peroneus are used interchangeably and are both considered correct.
- The short (brevis) digital extensor is a small muscle located on the dorsal side of the hock. Its tendon merges with the tendon of the long digital extensor.

Caudomedial Muscles of the Leg (Crus)

- The caudomedial muscle group of the leg includes the soleus, gastrocnemius, superficial digital flexor (SDF), deep digital flexor (DDF), and popliteus muscles.
- As a group, these muscles primarily function to extend the hock joint, with the exception of the popliteus, which plays a different role.
- Additionally, the SDF and DDF extend distally to help flex the digital joints. All of these muscles are innervated by the tibial nerve.
- The superficial digital flexor (SDF) in ruminants is more muscular compared to that of the horse, but it contains a tendinous band running through the muscle. In contrast, the SDF in the horse is predominantly tendinous.

Metatarsal

- **Two Metatarsals**

  a) Large (Fused 3rd and 4th metatarsals)

  b) Small (2nd metatarsal)

- **Large Metatarsal**

  a) Four Surfaces (Dorsal, Lateral, Medial and Plantar)

  b) Dorsal Vascular Groove (on dorsal surface)

  c) Proximal Interosseous Foramen

  d) Distal Interosseous Foramen

  e) Medial and Lateral Condyle, Sagittal Notch and Sagittal Ridge (Distal fExtremity)

  f) Facet for Small Metatarsal (on the medial surface, near proximal extremity)

Large Metatarsal (Dorsal View)

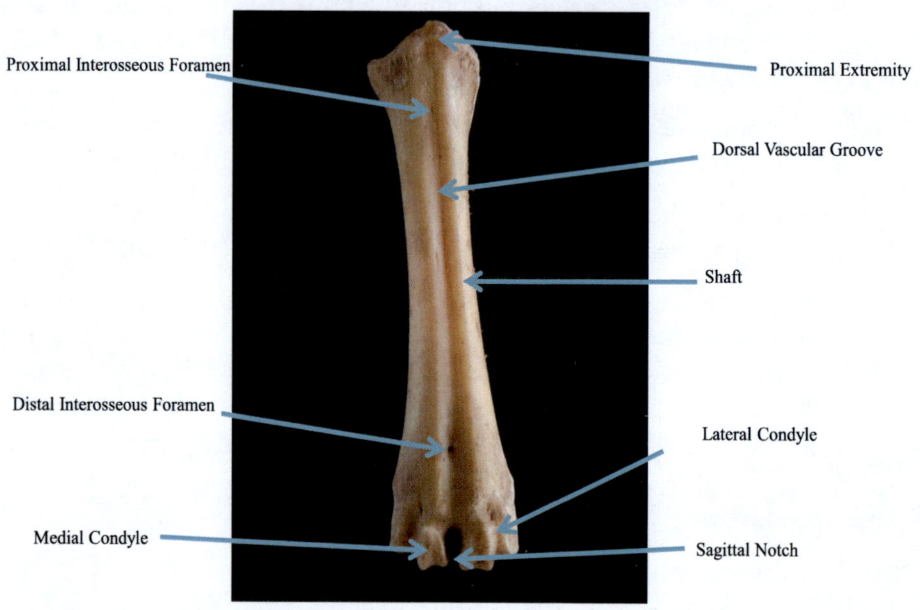

Instability of the fetlock

- Instability of the fetlock during weight bearing—such as flexion or knuckling—can be caused by spinal injuries resulting from trauma, like becoming trapped under the sides of a free stall, or from conditions such as spinal lymphosarcoma.
- Damage to the sciatic nerve, especially its peroneal branch, can also lead to fetlock knuckling. Additionally, painful conditions affecting the back of the foot, such as sole ulcers or severe digital dermatitis, may cause the animal to shift its weight forward onto the toe, resulting in knuckling. Therefore, it's essential to thoroughly examine the foot for any lesions that could contribute to this presentation.

Large Metatarsal (Plantar View)

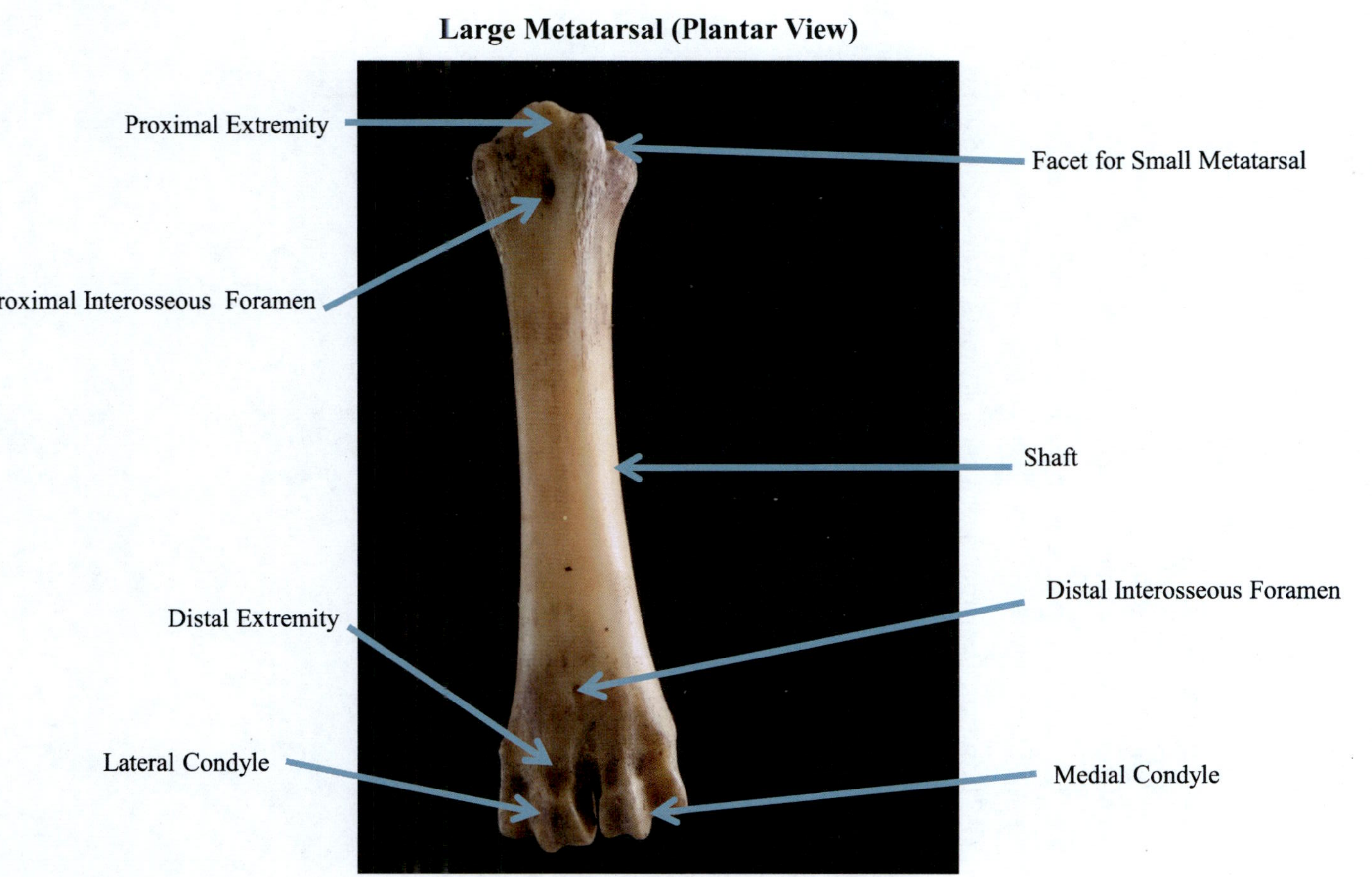

The common calcanean (Achilles) tendon and capped hock

- The common calcanean (Achilles) tendon is primarily formed by the tendons of the gastrocnemius and superficial digital flexor (SDF) muscles. Additional contributions come from the soleus, gluteobiceps, and semitendinosus muscles.
- At the point where these tendons insert on the calcanean tuber (the point of the hock), two types of bursae may be present:
- The subtendinous calcanean bursa, located between the gastrocnemius and SDF tendons, is a normal anatomical structure.
- The subcutaneous calcanean bursa is usually acquired and forms beneath the skin due to repeated friction against hard surfaces.
- In horses, inflammation of the subcutaneous calcanean bursa can cause a noticeable swelling at the point of the hock, a condition commonly referred to as "capped hock."

Large metatarsal (medial view)

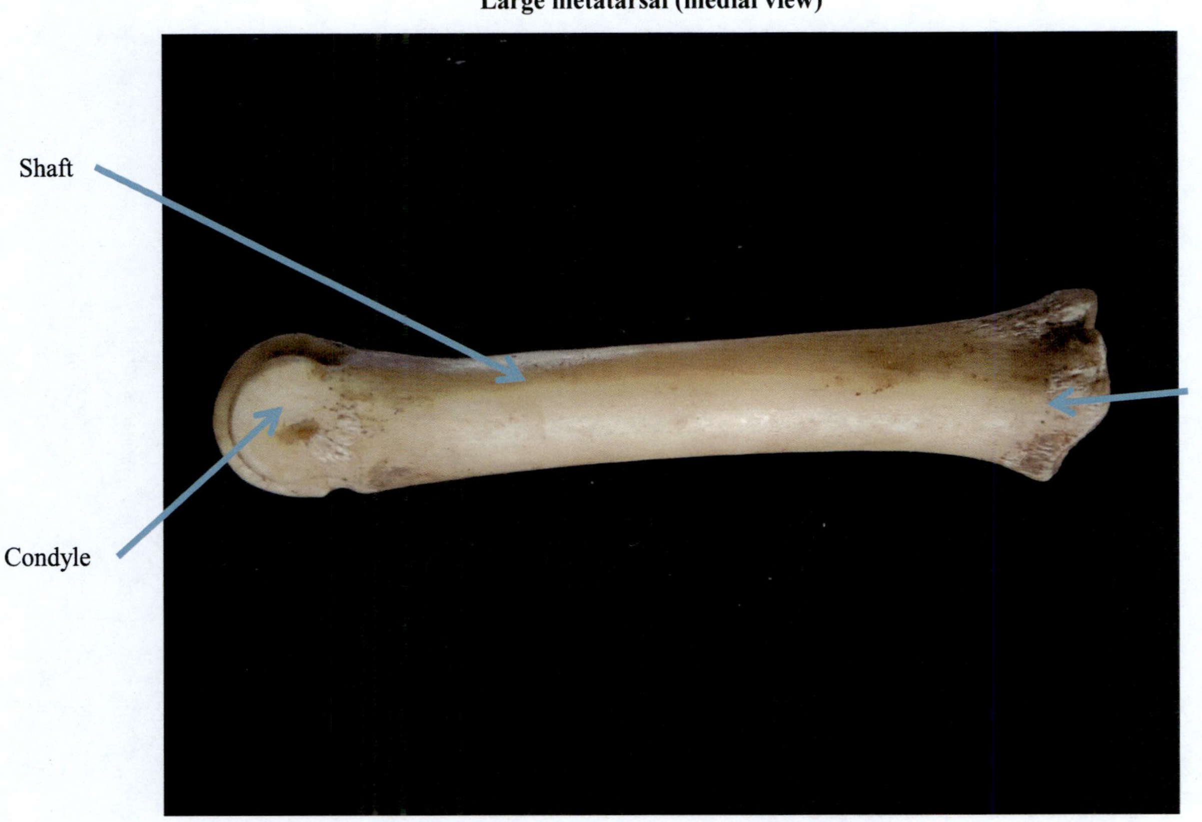

Superficial veins of the hindlimb

- The superficial veins of the hindlimb play a key clinical role in administering antibiotics or anesthetics—particularly for retrograde anesthesia targeting the distal foot.
- The cranial branch of the lateral saphenous vein, along with its branches (such as the dorsal common digital vein III or the lateral plantar digital vein), are commonly utilized for these procedures.
- When anesthetic is injected into these veins, it diffuses into the surrounding tissues and anesthetizes the digital nerves, enabling surgical interventions on the digits.

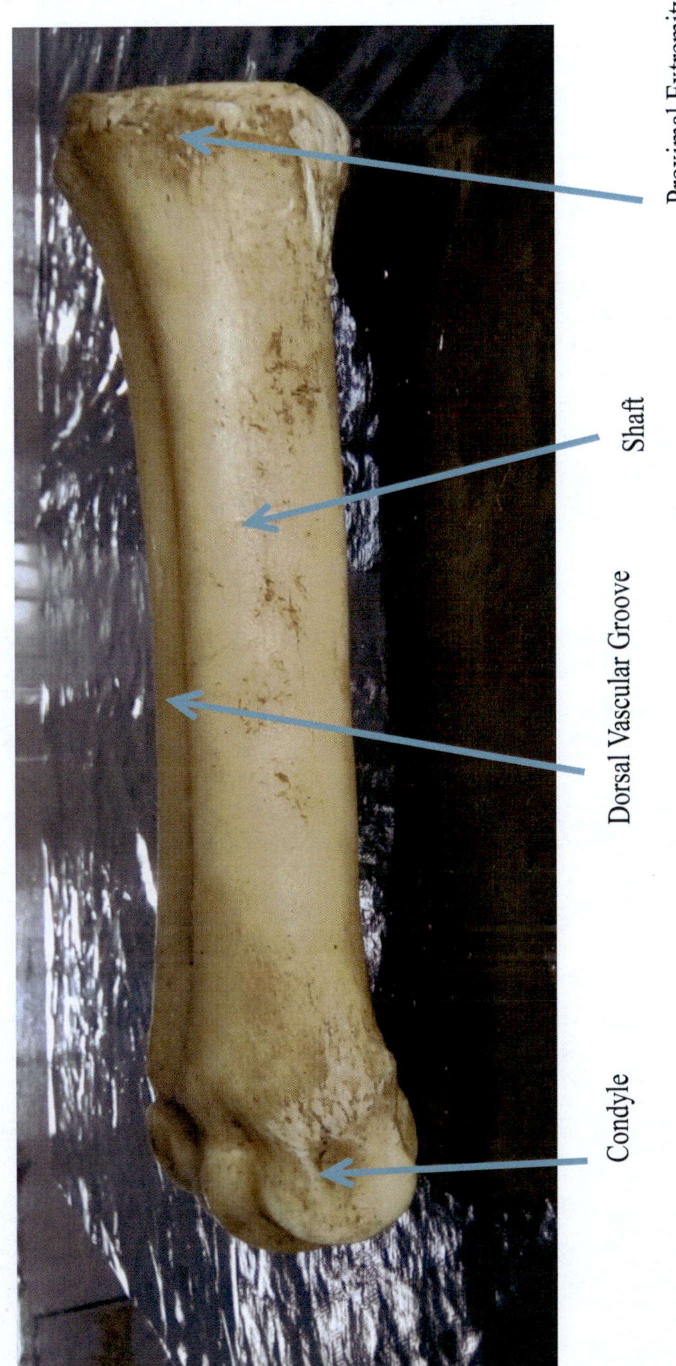

Large metatarsal (lateral view)

Sole hemorrhages and Sole ulcers

- Sole hemorrhages commonly develop beneath the flexor tuberosity of the third phalanx (P3) or along the white line, though they can appear anywhere on the weight-bearing surface of the hoof.
- The degree of lameness they cause depends on both the size of the hemorrhage and how long it has been present. These lesions should be regarded as early warning signs, potentially progressing to more serious hoof conditions like sole ulcers.
- Sole ulcers are areas of damage or penetration in the sole horn, caused by excessive pressure and repeated compression of the corium. They typically develop beneath the flexor tuberosity of the third phalanx (P3) and are often linked to varying degrees of pain and altered weight-bearing behavior.

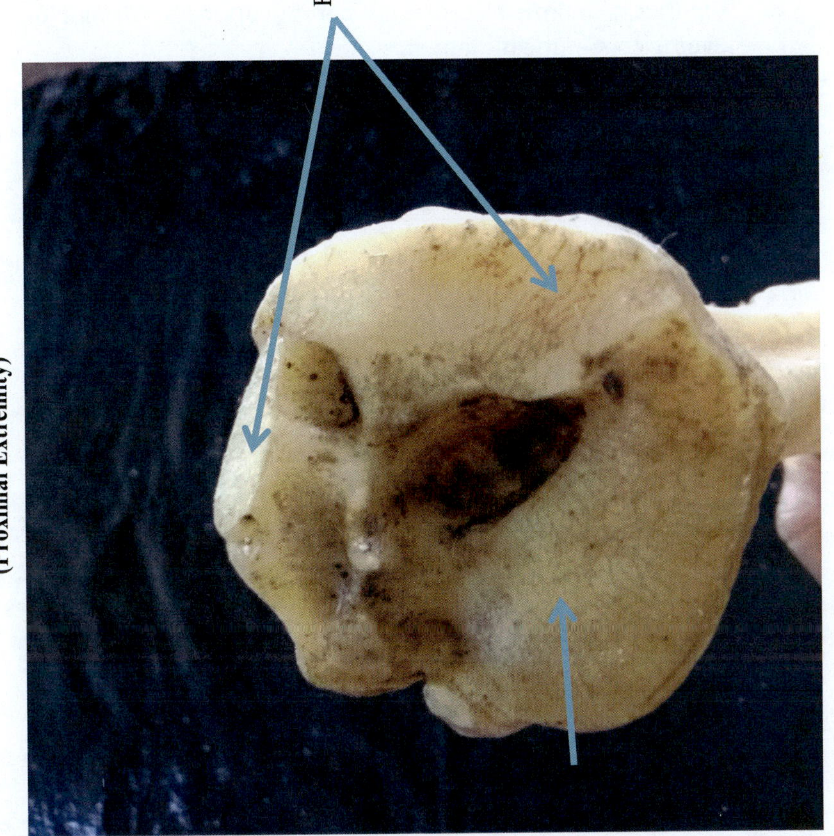

Large Metatarsal (Proximal Extremity)

Clinical conditions related to hoof in cattle-I

- **Deep digital sepsis** is a foot infection that affects the deeper structures, usually involving the distal interphalangeal joint and flexor tendons. This condition can develop as a rare complication following injuries such as foot rot, sole ulcers, or white line disease.
- **Thin sole** lesions develop when the sole horn has worn down sufficiently for the sole to flex under digital pressure, without exposing the corium.
- **Toe ulcers** and **toe necrosis** are complications resulting from thin soles, leading to significant lameness.
- **White line disease** refers to a variety of lesions, including hemorrhages, fissures, separations, and abscesses, that develop in the white line area.

Large Metatarsal (Distal Extremity)

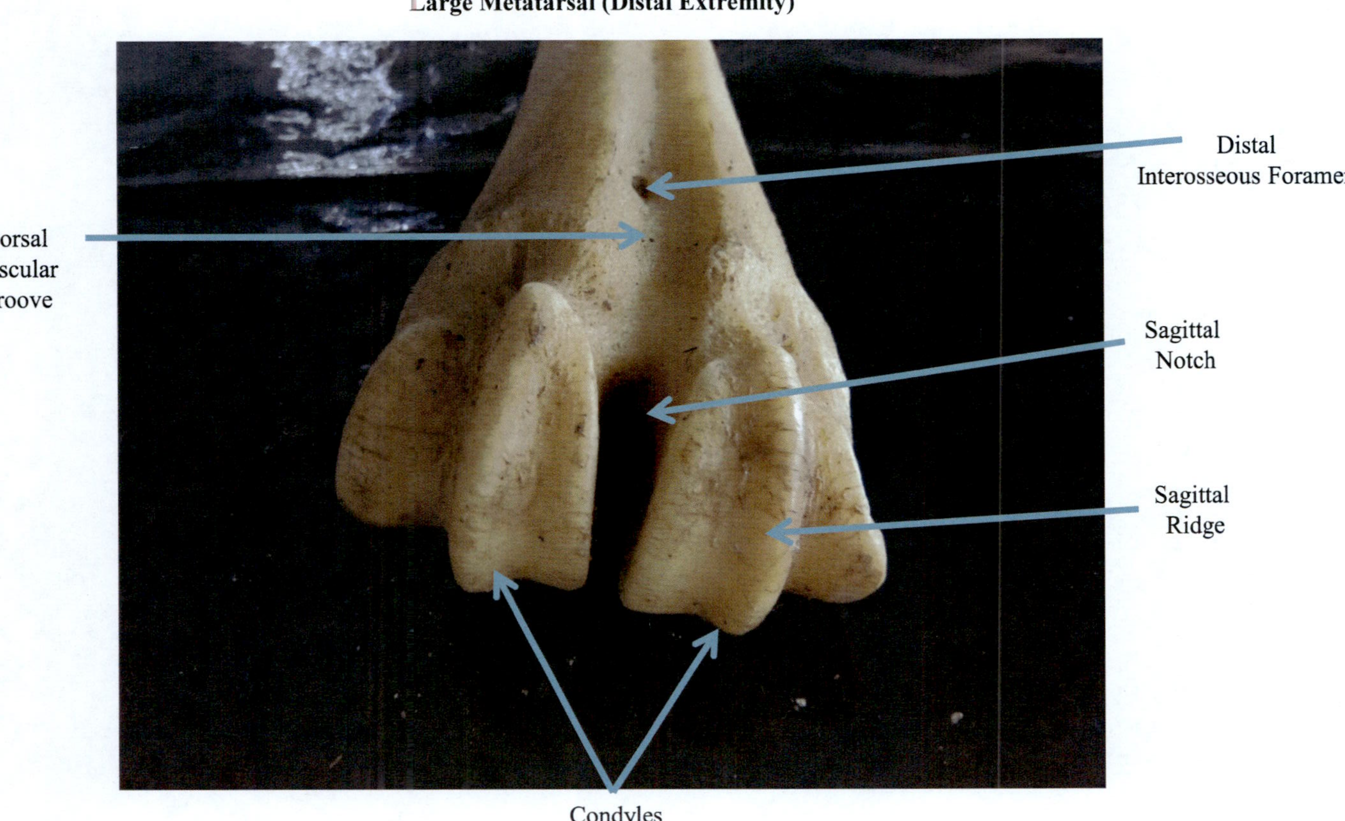

Clinical conditions related to hoof in cattle-II

- **A corkscrew claw** is a structural deformity of the phalanges seen in both beef and dairy cattle. While it was traditionally observed on the lateral claws of the hind feet in older animals, it is now increasingly found on the medial claws of both the front and hind feet in younger cattle as well.
- **Interdigital hyperplasia** refers to the excessive growth of fibrous tissue in the interdigital space of beef and dairy cattle.
- **The fissures** forming in the hoof walls, which may cause lameness if they extend into the corium. While fissures are rare in most herds, they can be classified based on their direction and location into horizontal, vertical, or axial wall fissures.

Large Metatarsal Plantar View (Proximal Extremity)

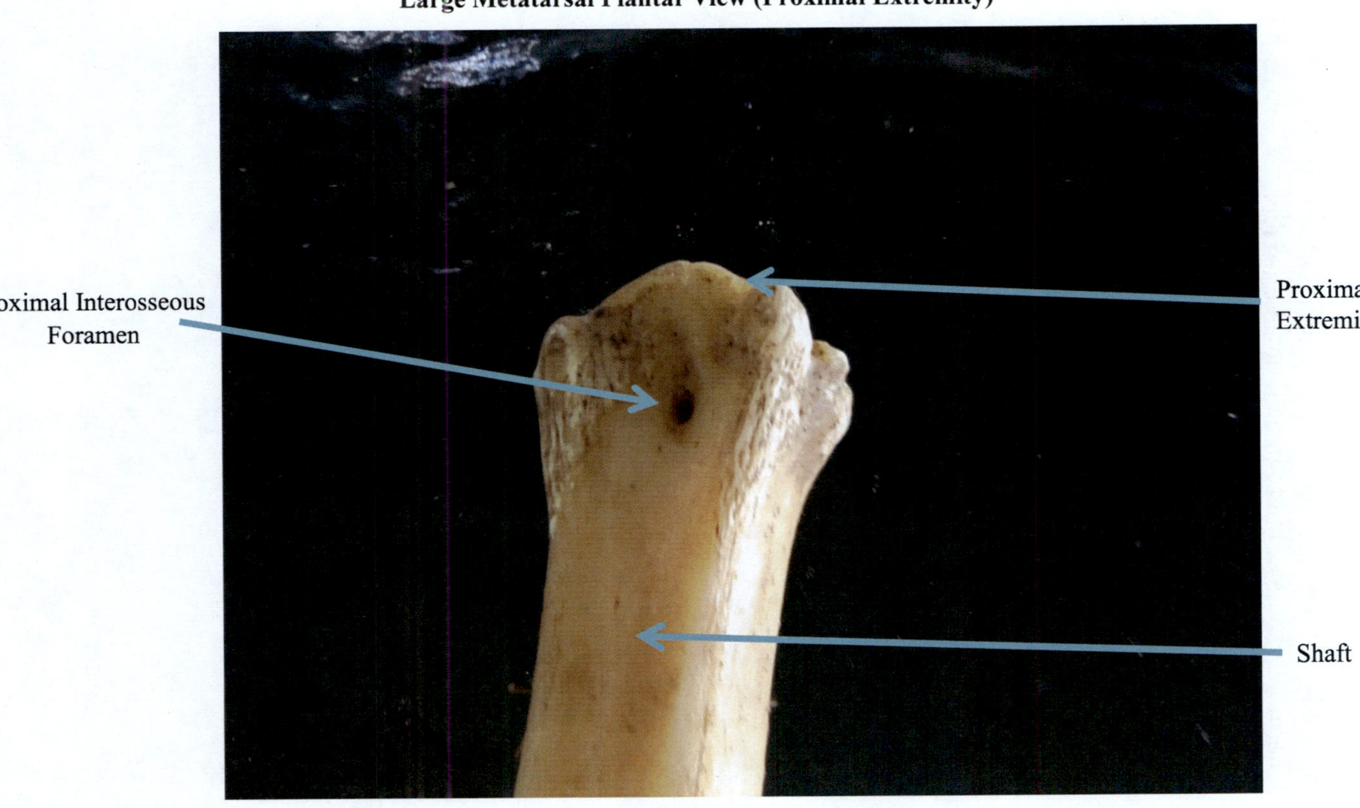

Hind limb becomes trapped or caught

- If a hind limb becomes trapped or caught, it can lead to hyperextension of the limb. As the animal attempts to free its foot, excessive tension may be placed on the fibularis tertius tendon, potentially causing it to rupture.
- A common clinical test to assess the integrity of this tendon involves flexing the stifle joint and observing the movement of the hock (tarsus).
- Under normal conditions, flexing the stifle prevents the hock from extending. However, if the fibularis tertius tendon is ruptured, the hock can be extended even when the stifle is flexed.

Axial Skeleton

- The axial skeleton is comprised of several key structures that form the central core of the animal skeleton.
- This includes the bones of the skull, which encase and protect the brain, the vertebral column or spine, which provides support and houses the spinal cord, as well as the ribs and the sternum, which together form the rib cage, protecting vital organs such as the heart and lungs.
- These components work together to provide structural support and protection for the body's central organs.

Skull Bones

The skull is a complex structure that varies greatly across different animal species, reflecting their unique evolutionary adaptations, dietary habits, and ecological niches.

Generally, the skull serves several critical functions: protecting the brain, supporting facial structures, and providing attachment points for muscles involved in feeding and expression.

Key Features of Animal Skulls

Cranium: This is the portion of the skull that encloses and protects the brain.

Facial Bones: These bones form the face and include the nasal bones, maxilla (upper jaw), and mandible (lower jaw).

Zygomatic Arch: This is the bone structure that forms the cheekbone and provides attachment for the muscles used in chewing.

Sutures and Fontanelles: Skull bones are connected by sutures—joints that allow for growth and, in some cases, slight movement. Fontanelles, or "soft spots," are gaps in the skull of young animals that eventually close as they mature.

Skull

- **Cranial bones**

  a) Frontal (considered to be present in the interface of cranial and facial bones)

  b) Parietal

c) Interparietal (paired in young animals, fused to a single bone in adult)

d) Occipital

e) Sphenoid

f) Ethmoid

g) Temporal

- Occipital, sphenoid and ethmoid are unpaired.

- **Facial bones**

a) Nasal

b) Pre-maxilla

c) Maxilla

d) Palatine

e) Lacrimal

f) Malar

g) Turbinate

h) Mandible

i) Hyoid

j) Vomer

k) Pterygoid

- Mandible, hyoid and Vomer are unpaired.

Skull

a) Frontal bone (determines the breed characteristic feature of the face)

- Cornual processes (horn)
- Supra orbital processes
- Supra orbital foramen
- Orbital plate
- Frontal suture (suture serrata)
- Torus frontalis

b) Parietal

- Caudal part
- Lateral part

c) Interparietal

- Placed in between the parietals.

d) Temporal bone

- Two parts: squamous and petrous part
- External Acoustic Meatus
- External Auditory Process
- Zygomatic Process of Temporal
- Tympanic bulla
- Condyle for the mandible
- Glenoid cavity
- Post glenoid process
- Post glenoid foramen
- Stylo mastoid foramen
- Internal Acoustic Meatus in the petrous part.

e) Occipital bone

- Supra occipital
- Lateral part
- Basi occipital
- External Occipital Protuberance
- Condyle
- Paramastoid process
- Condyloid fossa
- Basilar tubercle
- Foramen Magnum
- Foramen lacerum

f) Ethmoid

- Cribriform plate
- Crista galli
- Ethmoidal fossa
- Lateral Masses
- Perpendicular plate

g) Sphenoid

- Post sphenoid
- Body
- Temporal wings
- Foramen ovale
- Sella turcica
- Caudal clinoid process
- Pre sphenoid
- Body
- Orbital wings
- Foramen orbito rotundum

h) Premaxilla

- Nasal process
- Palatine process
- Incisive fissure
- Palatine fissure

i) Palatine bone

- Horizontal part
- Vertical part
- Cranial palatine foramen
- Caudal palatine foramen
- Spheno-palatine foramen

j) Lacrimal

- Lacrimal bulla

k) Maxilla

- Body
- Palatine process
- Zygomatic process
- Facial tuberosity at the level of 3rd cheek tooth
- Infra orbital foramen

l) Turbinate

- Dorsal turbinate
- Ventral turbinate

m) Malar bone (Zygomatic bone)

- Supraorbital process/ frontal process
- Zygomatic process/ temporal process

n) Nasal bone

- Nasal suture (suture harmonia)

o) Mandible

- Body
- Horizontal ramus
- Vertical ramus
- Angle
- Mandibular foramen medially
- Mental foramen laterally
- Condyle
- Coronoid process
- Mandibular notch

Characteristics features of skull of cattle

- In ruminants, the orbit forms a complete bony circle.
- In bovines, the facial crest is absent, replaced by a prominent bony structure known as the facial tuberosity.
- The temporal fossa is located caudal to the orbit and is relatively deep in bovines.
- At the rear edge of the bovine skull, there are two cornual processes that project from the frontal bone and form the bony bases of the horns.
- These processes are not found in polled animals, which are bred for this trait.
- In horned bovines, the cornual processes are hollow because the frontal sinus extends into them. The horn sheath covers the cornual processes.

Skull (Lateral View)

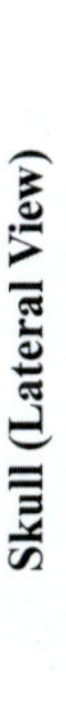

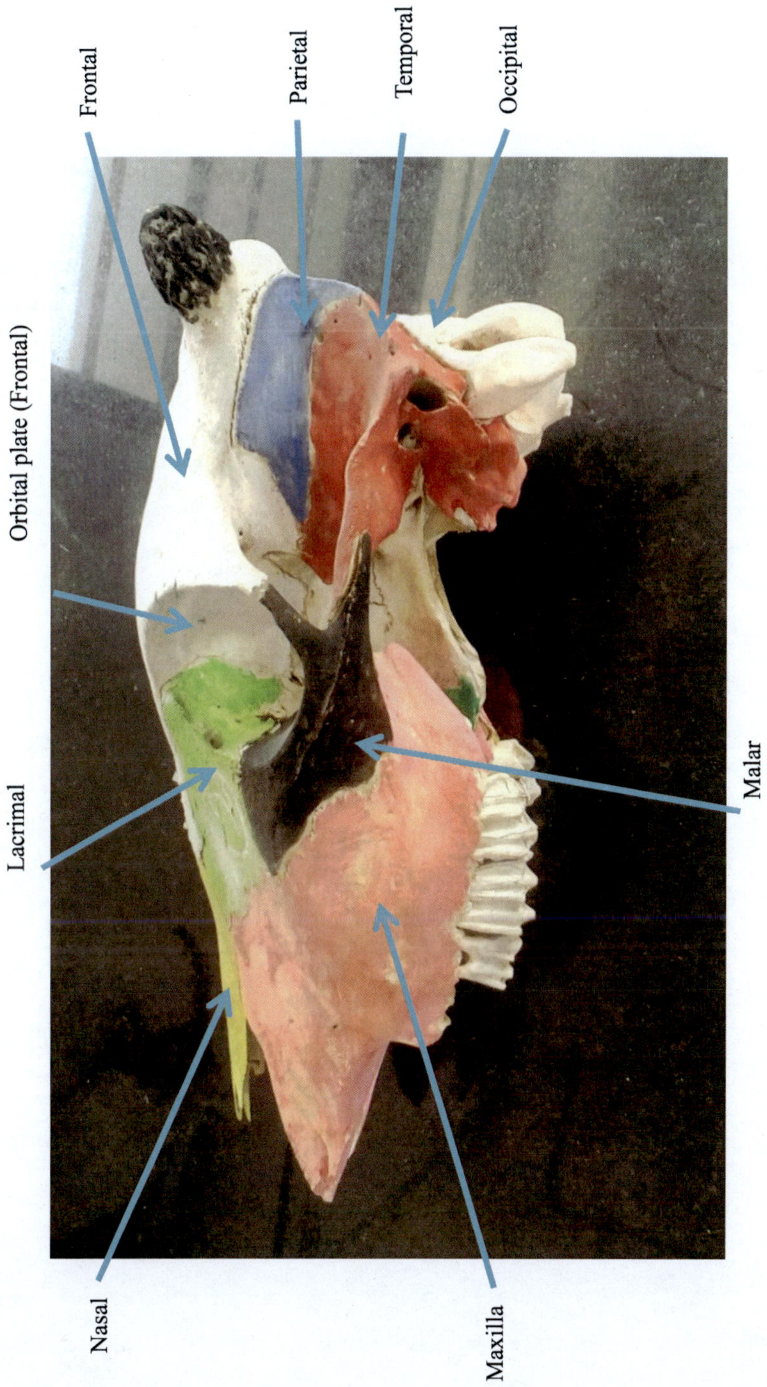

Important foramen/canal present in skull of cattle and nerve passes through it

Foramen/Canal	Nerve passes
Supraorbital foramen	Supraorbital nerve (branch of the ophthalmic division of the trigeminal nerve
Infraorbital foramen	Infraorbital nerve (maxillary division of the trigeminal nerve)
Mental foramen	Mental nerve (mandibular division of the trigeminal nerve)
Foramen orbitorotundum	Oculomotor nerve (III), trochlear nerve (IV), ophthalmic and maxillary division of the trigeminal nerve, (V) nerve and abducent nerve (VI)
Optic canal	Optic nerve (II)
Caudal palatine foramen	Major palatine nerve (maxillary nerve division of the trigeminal nerve)
Sphenopalatine foramen	Caudal nasal nerve (the maxillary nerve division of the trigeminal nerve)

Skull (Dorsal View)

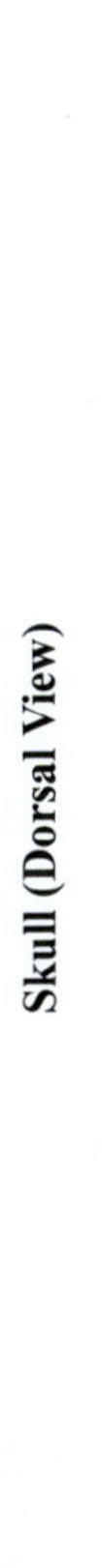

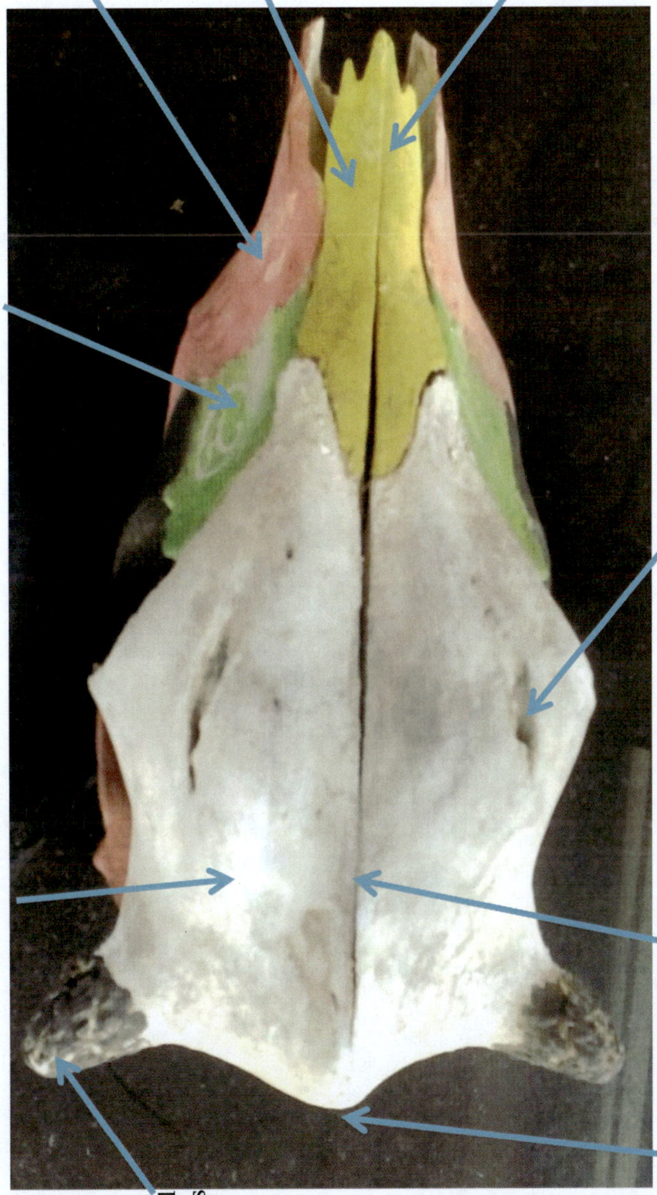

Horn buds: In order to inhibit the growth of horn buds, commonly referred to as horn buttons, in young animals, various procedures are employed. These methods include the application of chemical agents or heat cautery to prevent the development of the horns.

Dehorning in cattle: In dehorning procedures for cattle, the temporal line serves as a palpable landmark for blocking the cornual nerve, which is responsible for innervating the horn. Additionally, it is essential to ligate the cornual artery, which supplies blood to the horn, or alternatively, to cauterize its branches

Skull (Lateral View)

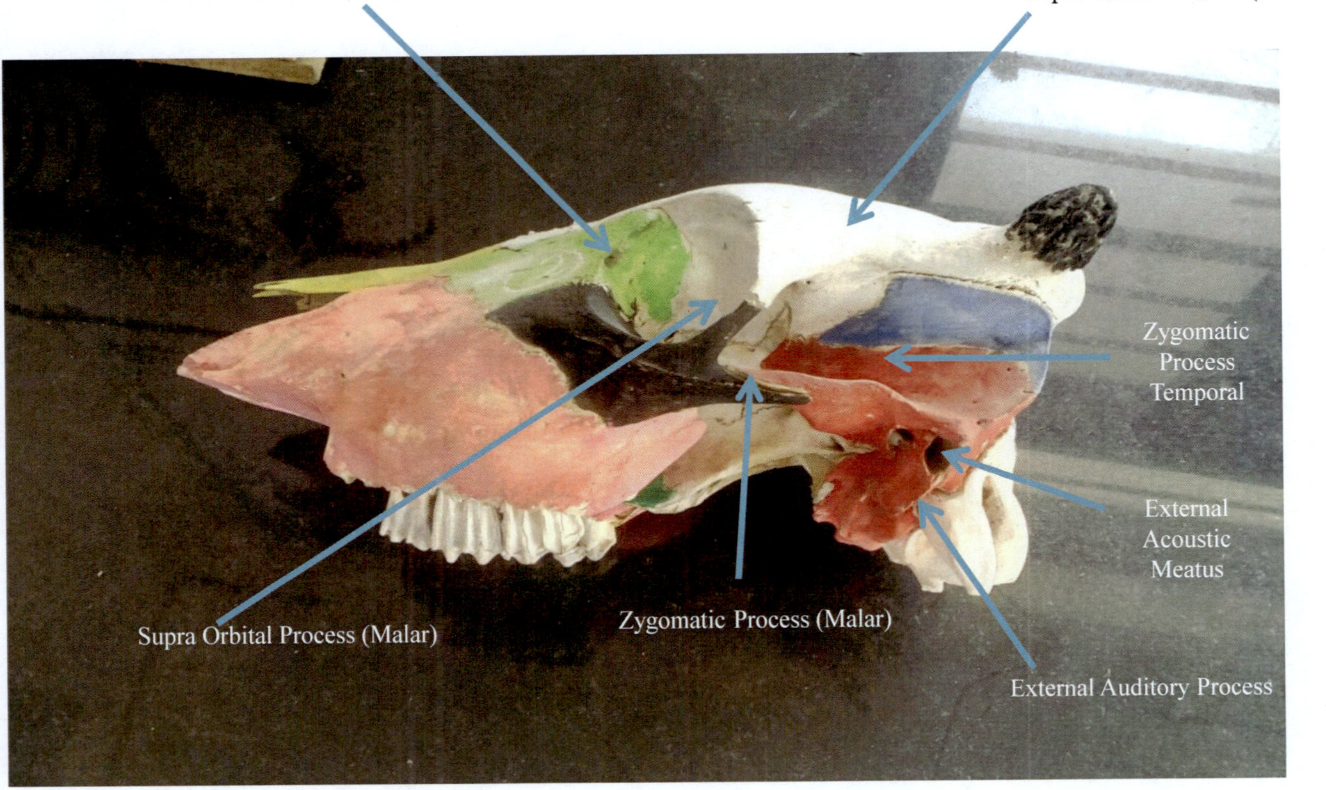

- The **zygomatic bone**, which constitutes the prominence of the cheek, delineates the boundary between the orbit and the temporal fossa.
- It establishes articulations with the maxilla, the greater wing of the sphenoid bone, as well as the zygomatic processes of both the frontal and temporal bones.
- The **external acoustic meatus (EAM)** is the auditory canal, a bony and cartilaginous structure that forms the passageway between the external ear and the middle ear.
- This canal serves as a conduit, transmitting sound waves from the outer ear to the tympanic membrane (eardrum) and subsequently to the middle ear.

Skull (Ventral View)

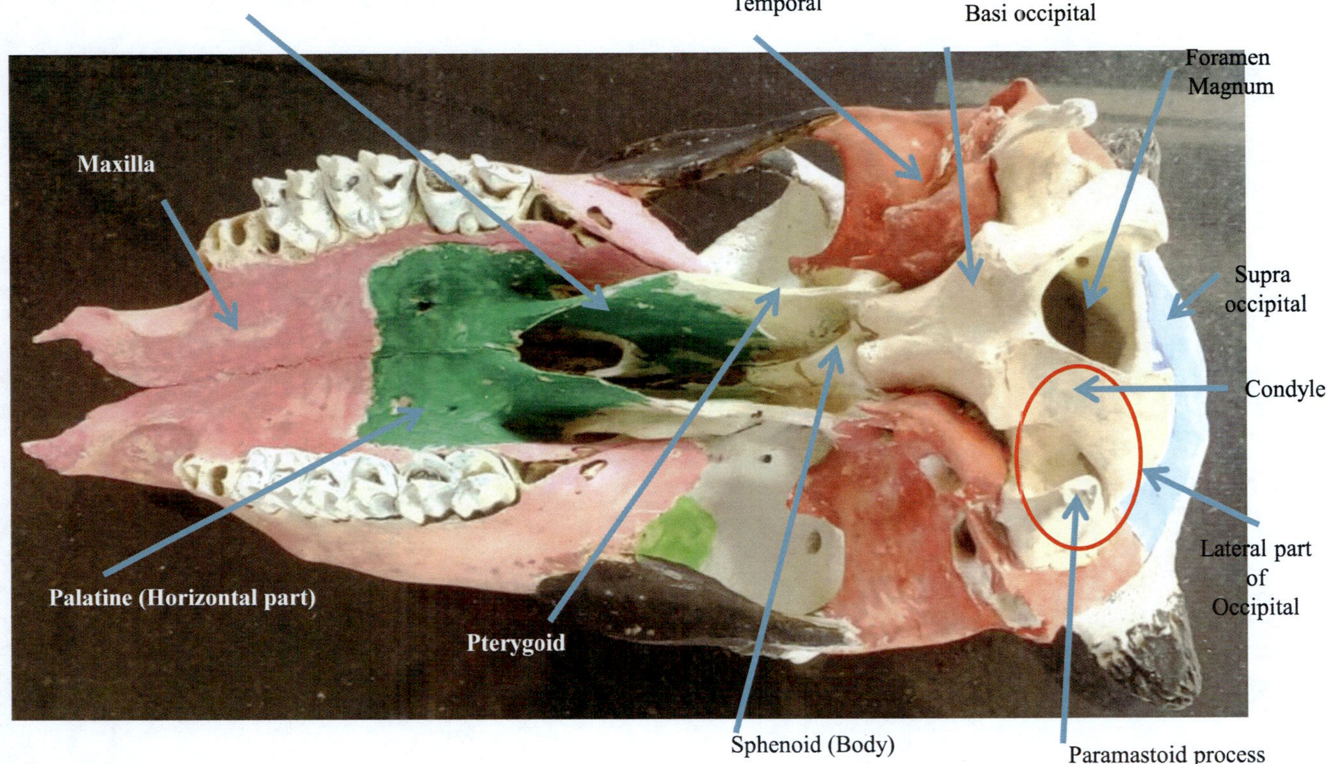

- **The hard palate** is primarily composed of the maxilla, although its posterior edge is formed by the palatine bone.
- **The soft palate** extends caudally from the hard palate and attaches to the margins of the palatine bone.
- In a mature specimen, there are six cheek teeth on each side of the bony palate.
- Dorsal to the hard palate lies the nasal cavity, while the nasopharynx is situated dorsal to the soft palate.
- Near the junction of the maxilla and palatine bones, there are prominent **palatine foramina**.
- These foramina allow for the emergence of the palatine artery, which supplies blood to the soft tissues of the palate.

Skull (Ventral View)

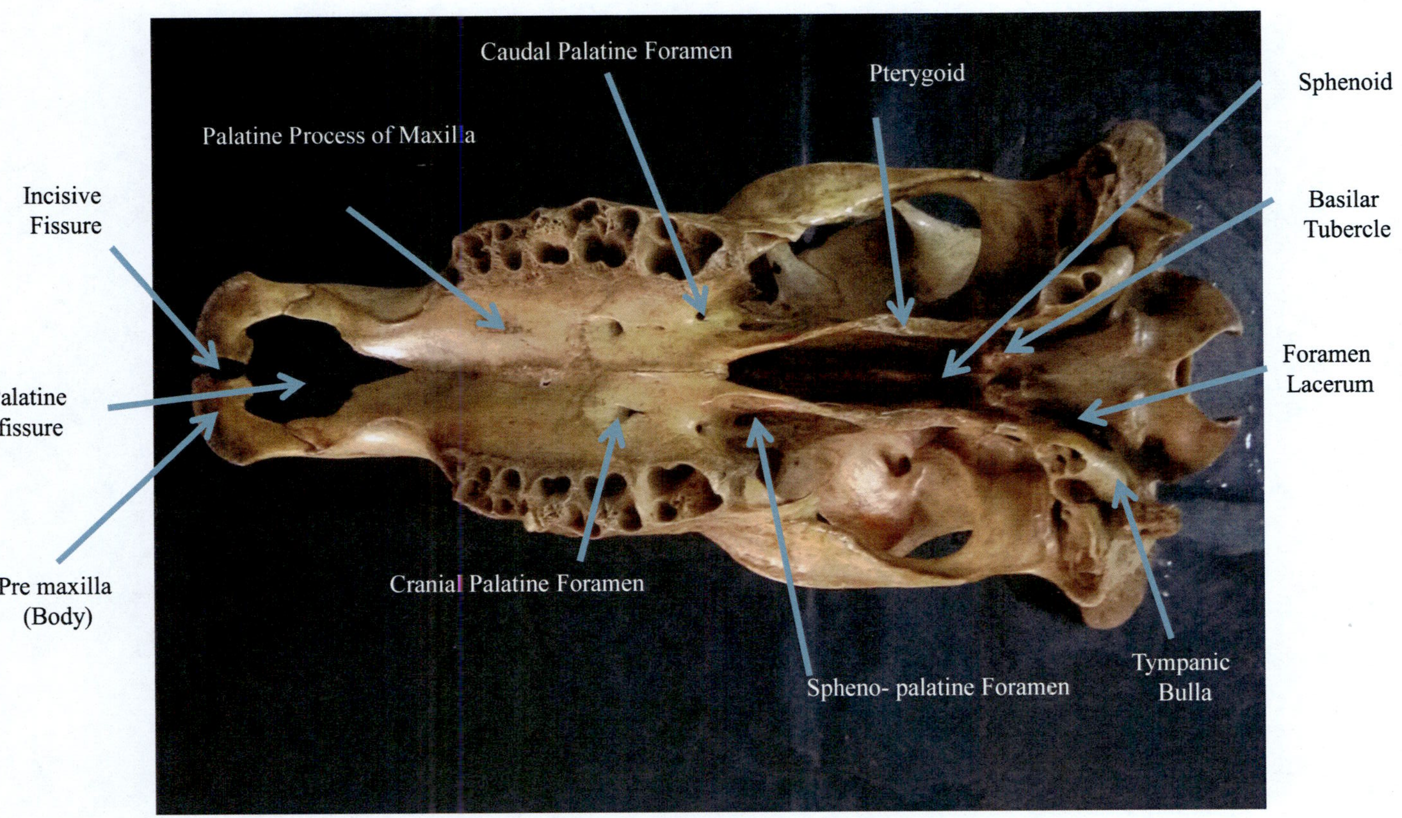

Clinical anatomy of horns in cattle

- Near the caudal and dorsal margins of the bovine skull, the cornual processes extend outward, forming the bony structure of the horn.
- These processes originate from the frontal bone; however, they are absent in polled cattle, which are naturally hornless.
- In horned cattle, the cornual process is hollow, a feature attributable to the extension of the frontal sinus known as the cornual diverticulum. Consequently, trauma to the horn can lead to an exposed sinus due to this anatomical connection.
- The "torus frontalis" in cattle refers to a prominent bony structure on the frontal bone of the skull. It's more commonly known as the "frontal bone torus" or "frontal ridge" and is particularly notable in the skulls of certain bovine breeds.
- It is often more pronounced in bulls and mature cattle compared to cows.

Skull (Caudal View)

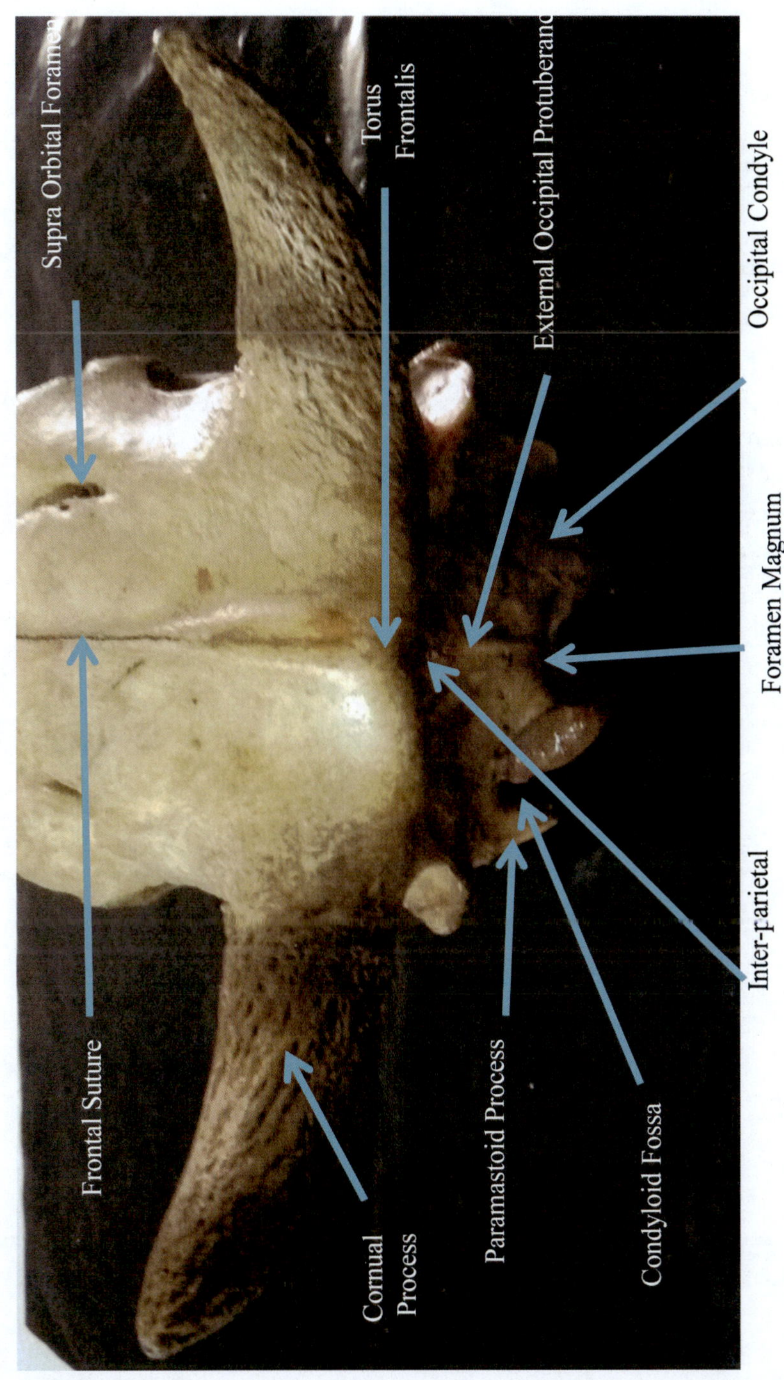

Nasal concha

- The nasal turbinates, also known as conchae, are paired structures consisting of thin-walled bony ridges that extend into the nasal cavity.
- The meatus refers to the passage or space located around each respective concha.
- Cattle have three main types of conchae: the dorsal nasal concha, the ventral nasal concha, and the ethmoidal concha.
- **Dorsal Nasal Concha:** Located towards the top of the nasal cavity, this concha is usually larger and less complex than the ventral one.
- **Ventral Nasal Concha:** This is a shorter and more prominent concha than horse that occupies the lower part of the nasal cavity. It has a more complex, scroll-like structure.
- **Ethmoidal Concha:** This concha is part of the ethmoid bone and is located further back in the nasal cavity. It is highly complex and contributes to the intricate structure of the nasal cavity.

Skull (Rostral View)

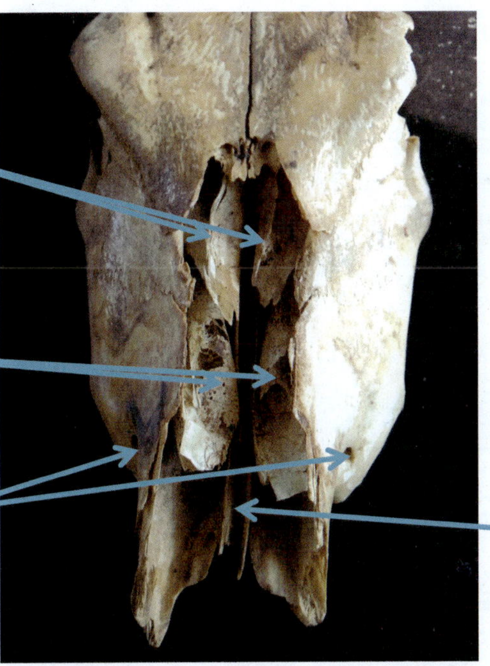

- The sphenoid bone in cattle is situated at the base of the skull and forms part of the **floor of the cranial cavity**.
- It is complex in shape and contributes to the formation of the orbit and the base of the skull.
- The ethmoid bone is located between the eyes and forms part of the medial wall of the orbit, as well as the **roof of the nasal cavity**.
- Its primary functions include supporting the nasal cavity and contributing to the structure of the orbit
- The internal acoustic meatus is a bony canal in the skull that allows the passage of nerves and blood vessels to the inner ear.
- In cattle, as in other mammals, this structure is important for hearing and balance.

Skull (Sagittal View)

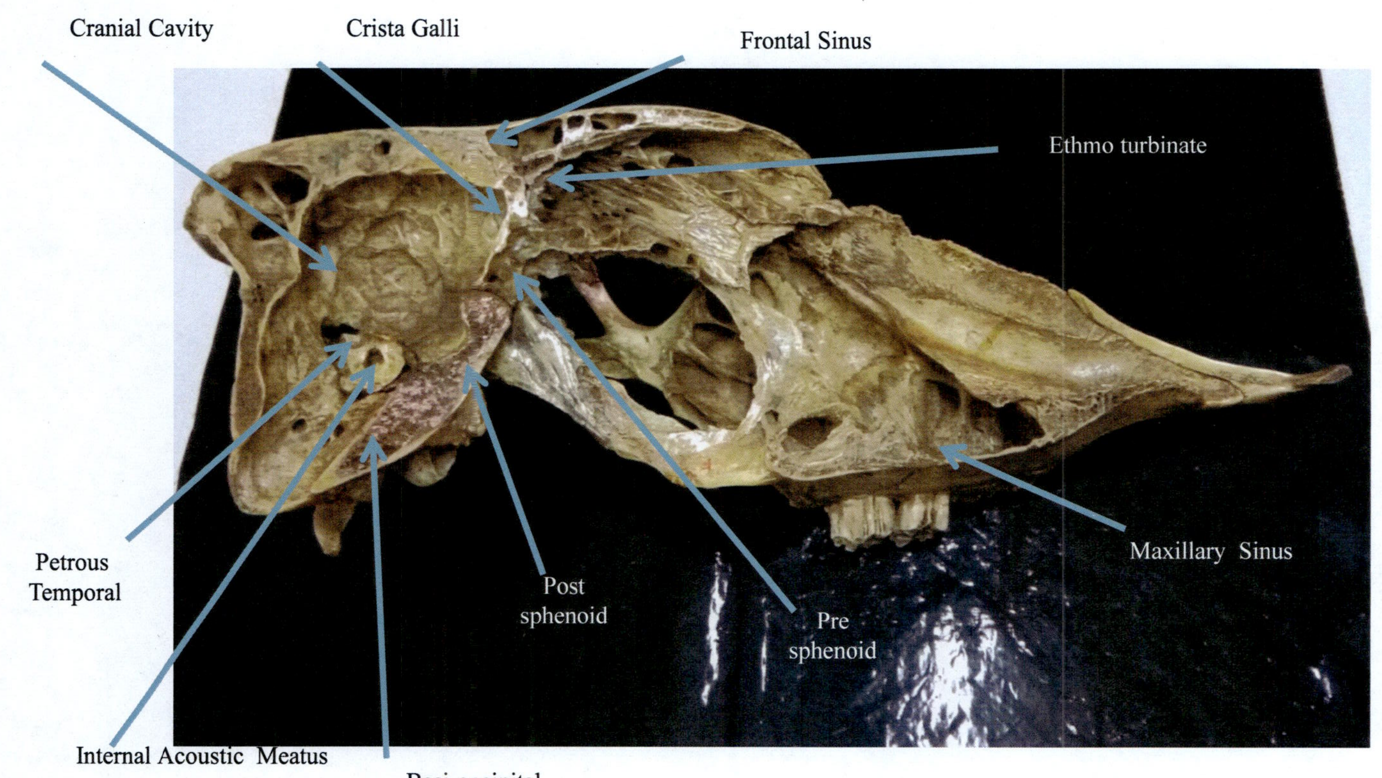

- **Optic Foramen (Optic Canal)**: Near the base of the skull, just in front of the sella turcica of the sphenoid bone. The optic nerve (cranial nerve II) and the ophthalmic artery pass through it.
- **Foramen Magnum**: The large opening at the base of the skull where the spinal cord exits the skull. The medulla oblongata, spinal cord, vertebral arteries, and spinal accessory nerves (cranial nerve XI) are the content.
- **Infraorbital Foramen**: On the maxilla, just below the eye socket. The infraorbital nerve (a branch of the maxillary nerve, cranial nerve V2).
- Understanding these foramina and their contents helps in diagnosing and managing various conditions in cattle, especially when dealing with neurological symptoms, trauma, or surgical planning.

Skull (Ventral View)

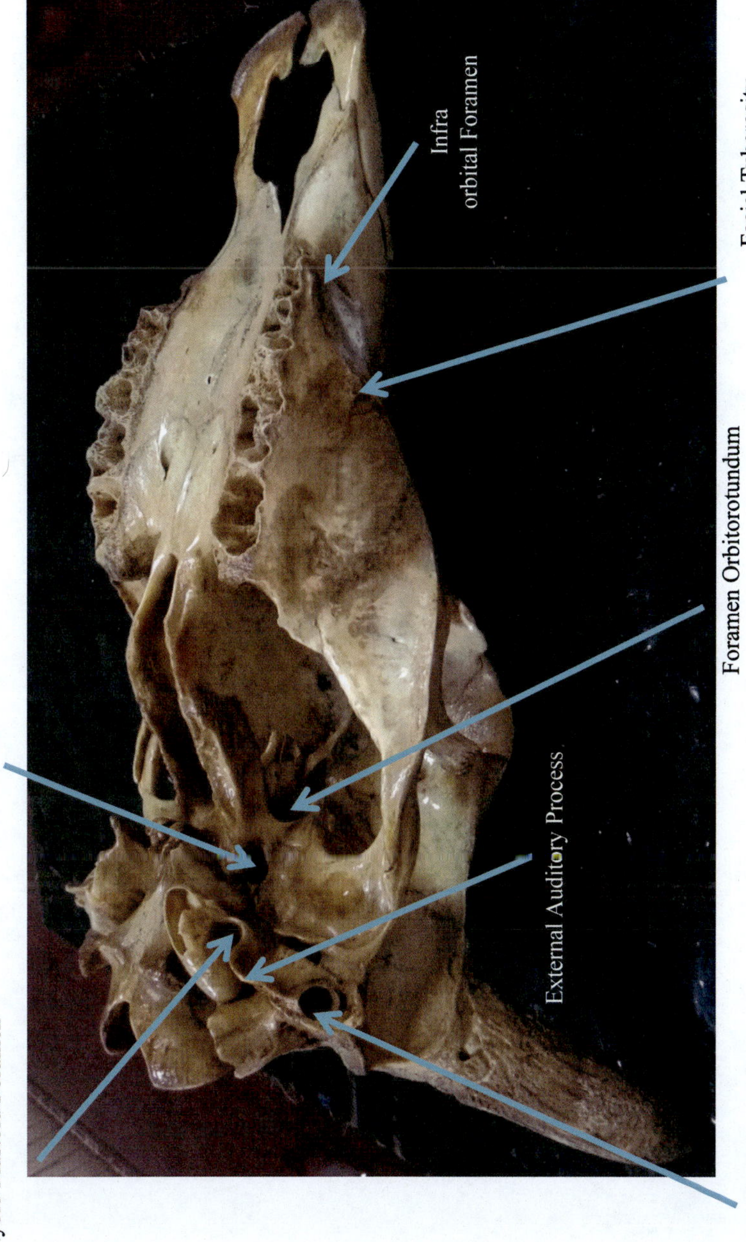

Temporomandibular joint

- In cattle, the mandible (lower jaw) attaches to the temporal bone (part of the skull) through a joint known as the temporomandibular joint (TMJ).
- This joint is crucial for the movement of the jaw, allowing the cattle to chew and move their mouth.
- The broad caudal section features a ventral surface that articulates with the mandibular condyle.
- This surface includes a transversely elongated condyle, with the glenoid cavity situated behind it.
- The fossa is bounded posteriorly by the postglenoid process, which has an articular cranial surface. Behind this process lies a fossa containing the postglenoid foramen, the external opening of the temporal canal.

Skull (Ventral View, Focussing area of mandible attachment)

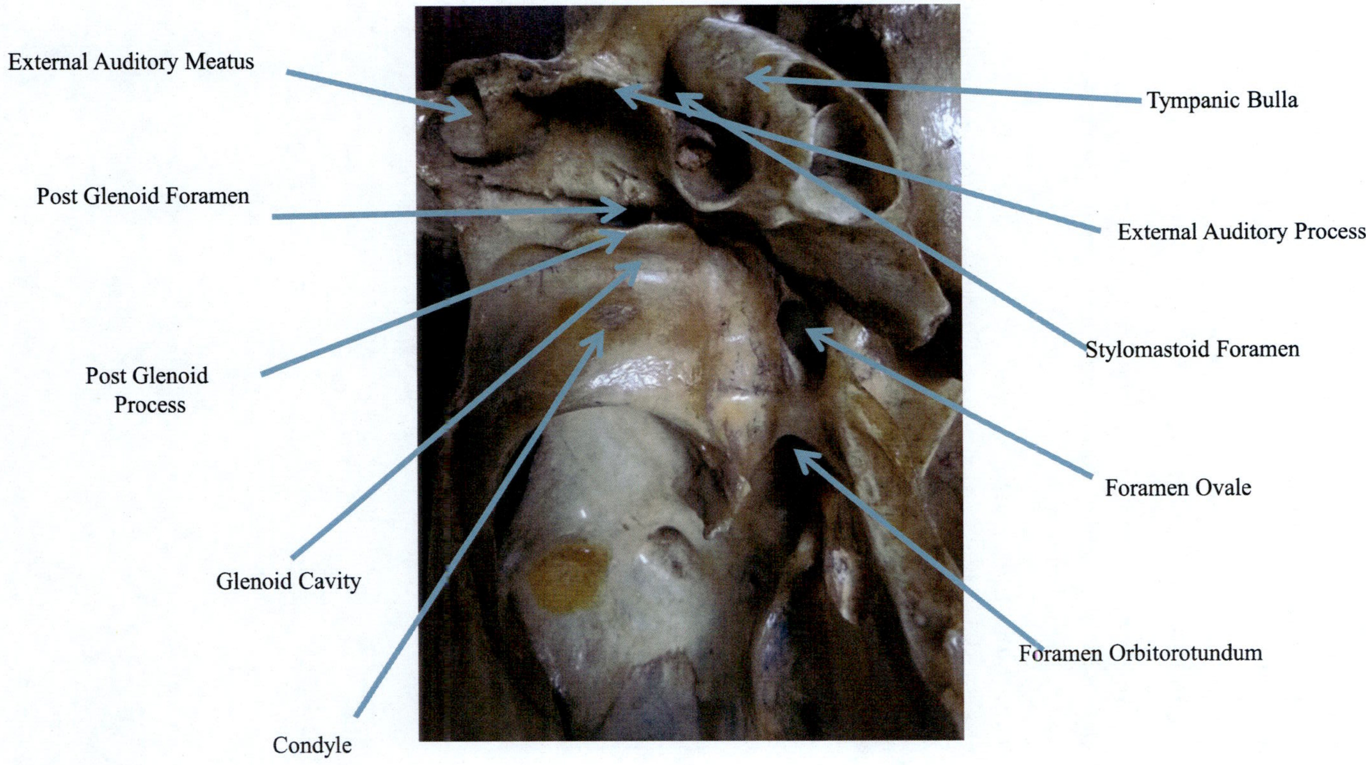

- The ethmoid bone in cattle, like in other mammals, is a complex structure that forms part of the skull. It's located in the front portion of the skull, between the eyes and forming part of the nasal cavity. The ethmoid bone is positioned between the frontal bones and the nasal bones.
- It helps separate the nasal cavity from the brain cavity and contributes to the formation of the orbit (eye socket).
- **Cribriform Plate:** This is a horizontal, perforated plate at the top of the ethmoid bone that allows the olfactory nerves to pass from the nasal cavity to the brain.
- **Ethmoidal Labyrinth:** Located on either side of the cribriform plate, these are complex structures of thin-walled cells that contribute to the nasal cavity's surface area and aid in the conditioning of inhaled air.
- **Perpendicular Plate:** This is a vertical plate that forms part of the nasal septum, helping to divide the nasal cavity into left and right halves.

Inner Side of the Cranial Cavity (Enlarged View)

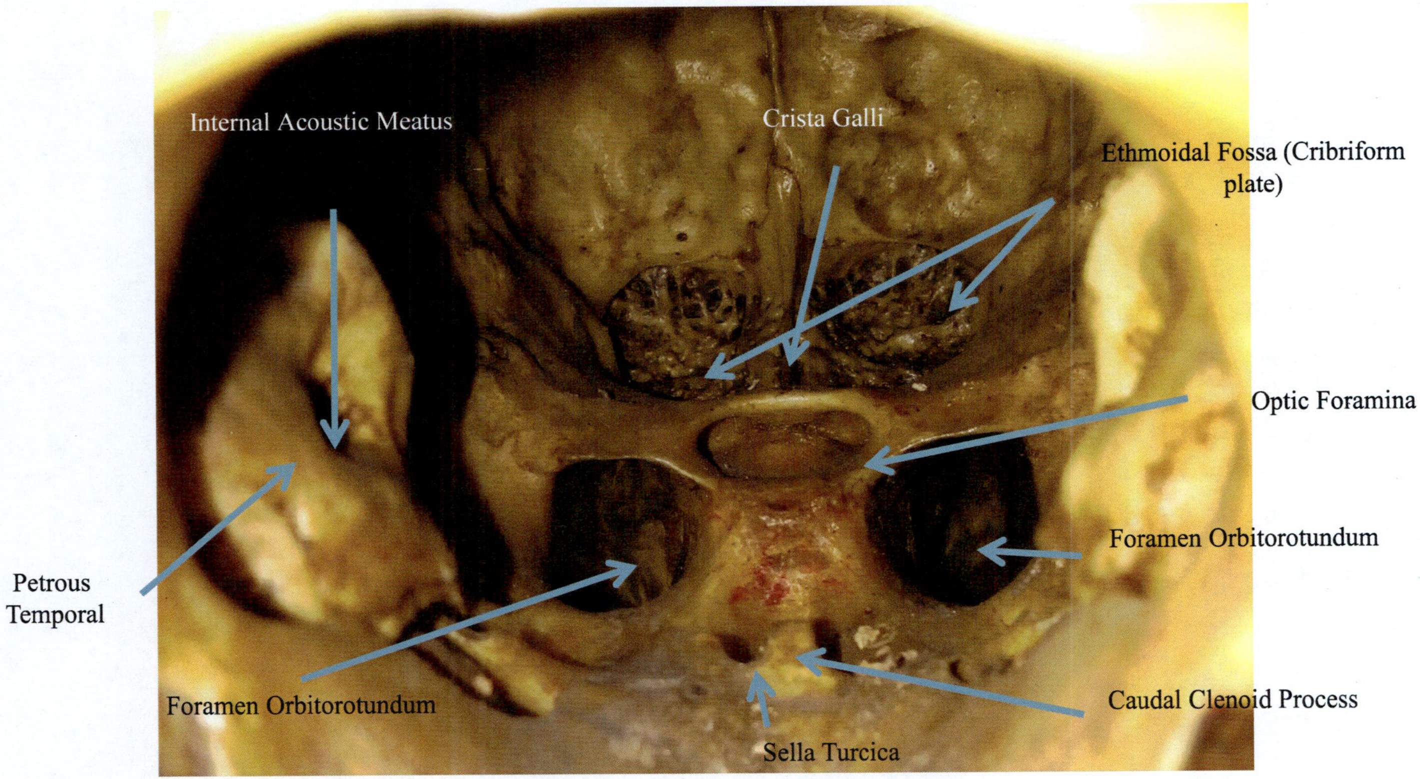

Internal Acoustic Meatus

Crista Galli

Ethmoidal Fossa (Cribriform plate)

Optic Foramina

Petrous Temporal

Foramen Orbitorotundum

Foramen Orbitorotundum

Caudal Clenoid Process

Sella Turcica

- **The mandible of cattle**, or the lower jaw, plays a crucial role in their anatomy, particularly in feeding.
- It consists of a body and two rami (horizontal and vertical ramus) that extend upward to connect with the skull at the temporomandibular joint.
- The junction of the horizontal and vertical ramus forms the angle of the mandible.
- On the proximal aspect of the vertical ramus, the coronoid process extends downward. The condylar process projects caudally from the ramus and articulates with the mandibular fossa of the skull, forming the temporomandibular joint (TMJ).
- The mandibular notch lies between the coronoid and condylar processes.

Mandible (Lateral View)

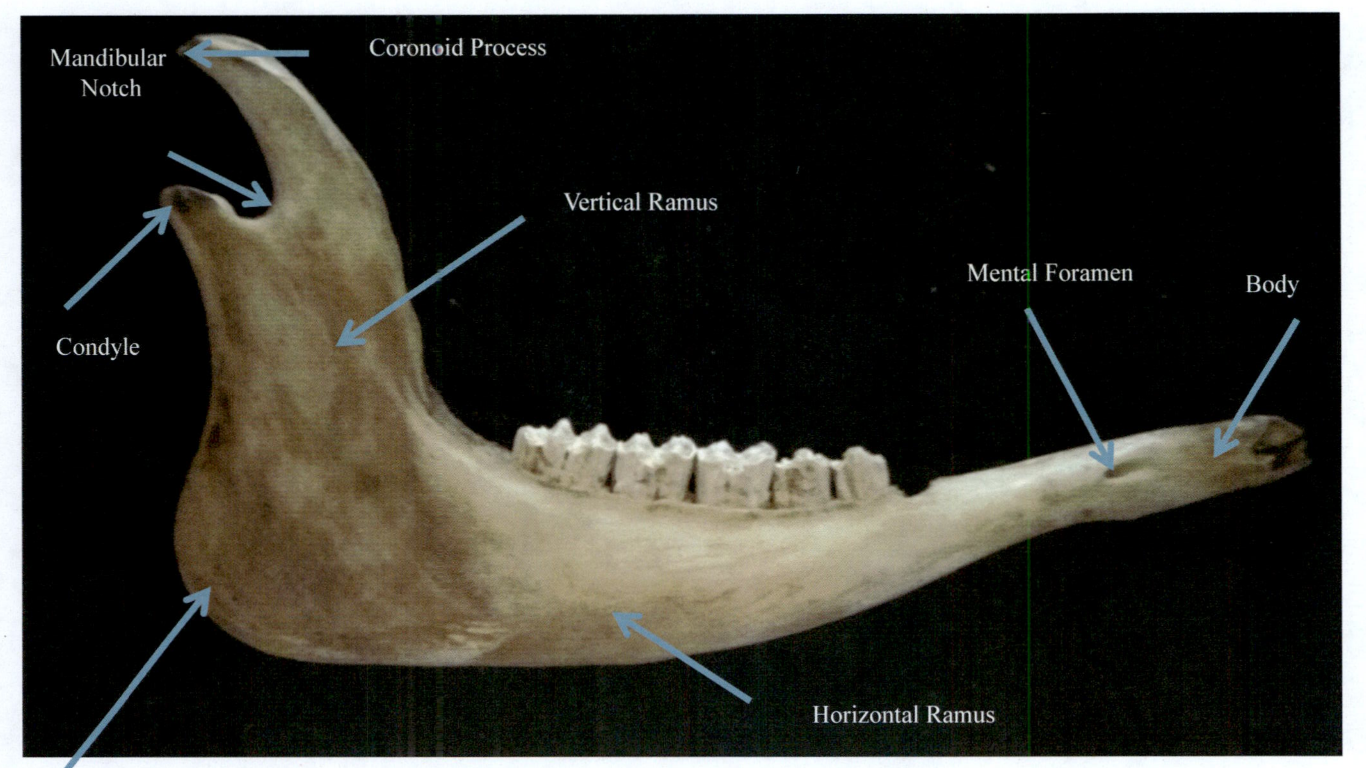

- On the medial side of the ramus lies the **mandibular foramen**, which serves as the entry point to the mandibular canal within the body of the mandible.
- **The inferior alveolar nerve** enters the mandibular foramen and travels through the mandibular canal, providing alveolar branches to the mandibular teeth. It then exits on the lateral surface as the mental nerve through the mental foramen.
- **The mandibular symphysis** in cattle is less robust than that of horses and undergoes ossification later in life. While mandibular fractures are uncommon in cattle, they can occur in young calves, particularly when their heads are manipulated with a snare.

Mandible (Medial View)

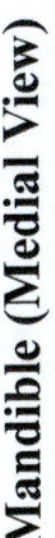

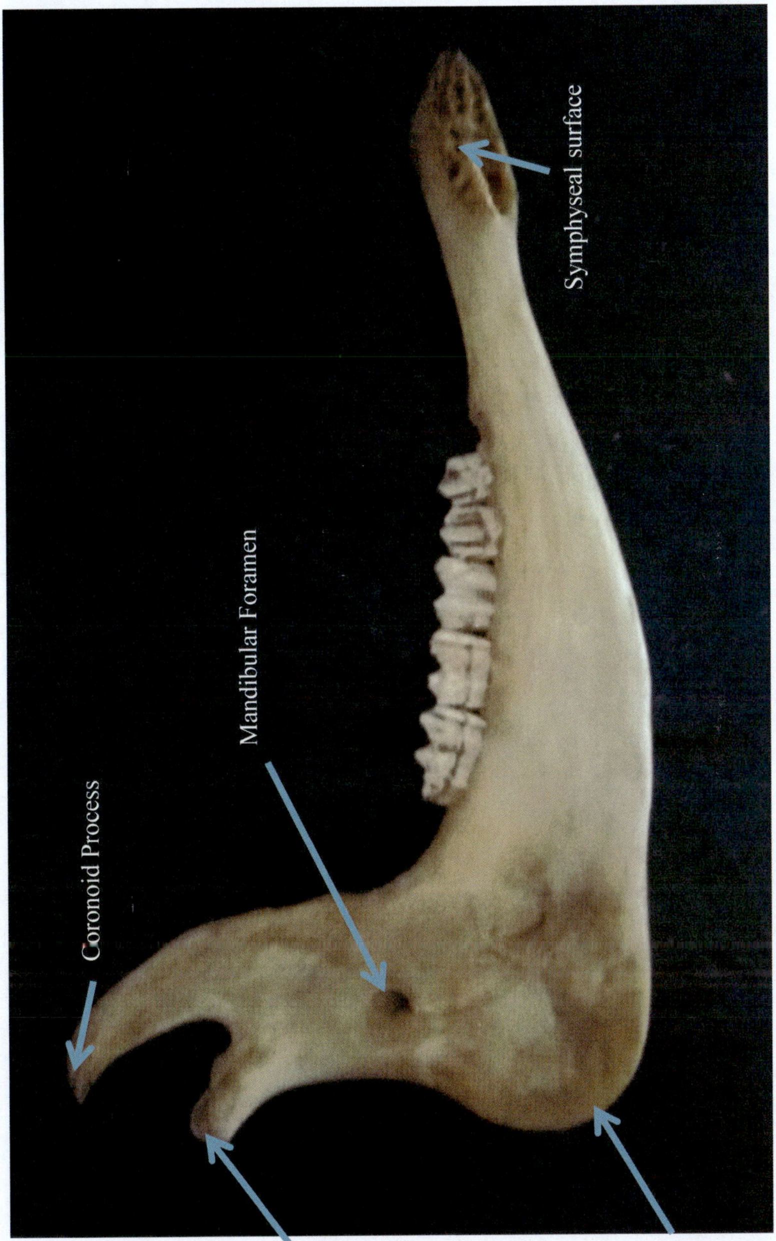

Paranasal Sinuses

- Paranasal sinuses are air-filled cavities located within the bones of the skull, surrounding the nasal cavity. They are lined with mucous membranes and play several important roles
- Cattle possess six paranasal sinuses: the frontal, maxillary, palatine, lacrimal, sphenoid, and conchal sinuses.
- Drilling a circular hole in the skull or other bones is called **trephination**. This procedure is typically performed to drain inflammatory fluid and to cleanse the sinuses with an antiseptic solution.
- The frontal sinus is quite extensive, encompassing nearly the entire frontal bone and a significant portion of the posterior wall of the cranium. It can also extend a varying distance into the comual processes when they are present.
- Diseases of the frontal sinus often arise from microbial infections, frequently linked to dehorning operations in cattle.

Vertebrae

- Vertebrae are the bones that make up the vertebral column (spine) in animals, providing support and protection for the spinal cord.
- The vertebral column is a key component of the skeleton, made up of a series of median, unpaired, irregular bones that extend from the skull to the tail.
- In adults, some vertebrae fuse together to create a single bony structure that connects with the pelvic girdle. These fused vertebrae are known as fixed (or false) vertebrae, in contrast to the movable (or true) vertebrae.
- The column is divided into five regions, each named after the corresponding part of the body where the vertebrae are located.
- These regions are referred to as cervical, thoracic, lumbar, sacral, and coccygeal. The vertebral formula is C-7 T-13 L-6 S-5 Cy-18-20.

Vertebra

- Body
- Arch
- Processes
  a) The articular processes
  b) The spinous process or spine
  c) The transverse processes
  d) Mammillary processes
  e) Accessory processes
  - The Cervical
  - The Thoracic
  - The Lumbar
  - The Sacrum
  - The Coccygeal

Cervical Vertebra

- Seven in number
- Typical Cervical Vertebra (3rd, 4th and 5th)

a) Cranial extremity (strongly convex)

b) Caudal extremity (strongly concave)

c) Transverse process divided in to dorsal and ventral parts

d) Ventral spine

- **Atypical Cervical Vertebra (Atlas, Axis, 6th and 7th)**

- **Atlas**

a) Body and spinous process absent

b) Wings

c) Lateral masses

d) Fovea dentis

e) Dorsal tubercle

f) Ventral tubercle

Cervical Vertebra

- **Axis**

a) Body

b) Dens or odontoid process

c) Very large spinous process

- **6th cervical**

a) Plate like ventral division of transverse process

- **7th Cervical**

a) Undivided spinous process

b) Spinous process resemble with thoracic vertebra

c) Costal facet on Caudal extremity of body

- Foramen transversarium (absent in Atlas and 7th)

Atlas (Dorsal View)

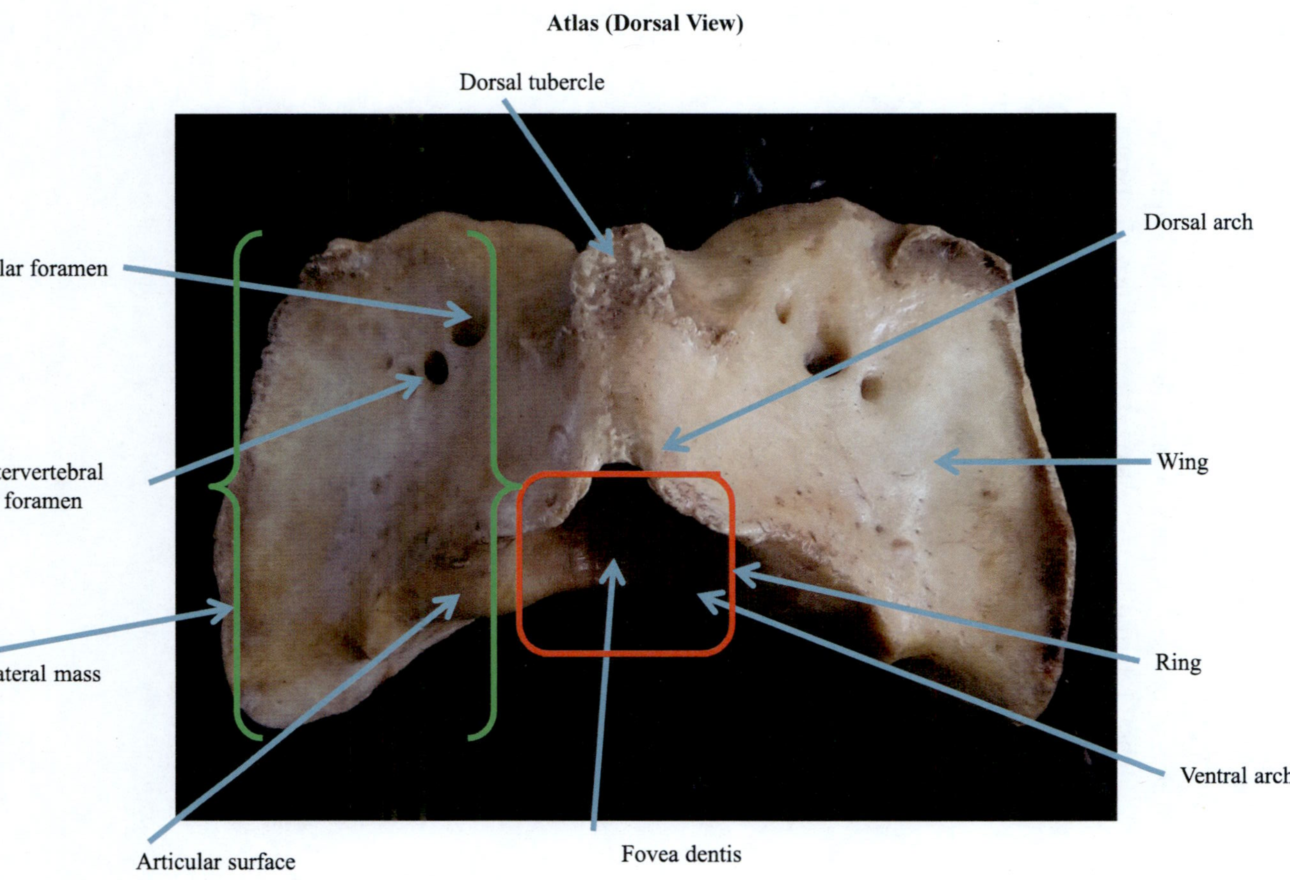

Cervical Vertebra

- It forms the skeleton of neck.
- The cervical vertebrae comprise seven distinct bones, categorized into typical and atypical types.
- The first cervical vertebra, known as the atlas, and the second cervical vertebra, referred to as the axis, are classified as atypical due to their unique anatomical features.
- The third, fourth, and fifth cervical vertebrae are considered typical, exhibiting similar structural characteristics. In these vertebrae, the transverse process is divided into two parts.
- However, in the sixth cervical vertebra, while similar in many respects, certain features begin to diverge.
- The seventh cervical vertebra is unique in that its transverse process is undivided, marking a notable distinction from the preceding vertebrae.
- This variation among the cervical vertebrae plays a crucial role in the overall functionality and mobility of the cervical spine.

Atlas (Ventral View)

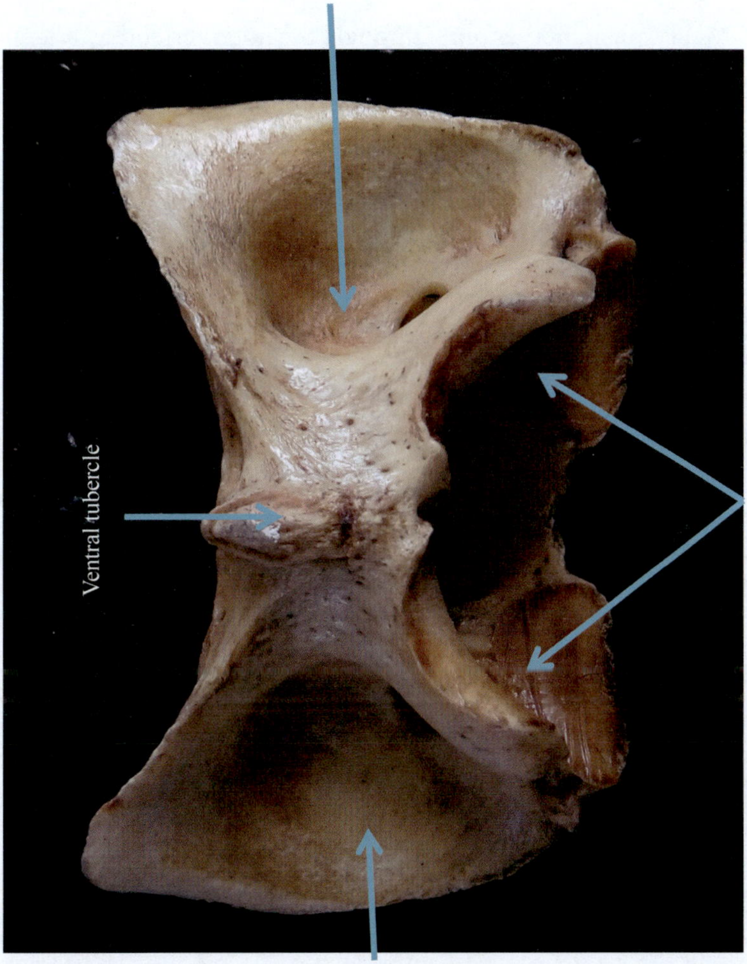

Ventral tubercle

Fossa atlantis

Articular cavities

Wing

Clinical conditions related to cervical vertebra

- Slight malformations or narrowing of the cervical vertebrae or the vertebral canal, frequently attributed to degenerative processes, can lead to spinal cord damage, manifesting as gait deficits commonly referred to as **Wobbler syndrome**. Additionally, symptoms may encompass restricted dorsiflexion of the neck, contingent upon the specific cervical region impacted.
- Most spinal nerves exit through the intervertebral foramina, located between adjacent vertebrae. However, the first two cervical vertebrae are an exception, as spinal nerves exit in different ways, including through lateral vertebral foramina.
- A laminectomy involves the partial or complete removal of a lamina. When disc material from the nucleus pulposus protrudes into the spinal cord, it can create pressure that disrupts nerve signals both upstream and downstream. This procedure is often performed to relieve pressure on the spinal cord.

Atlas (Craniodorsal View)

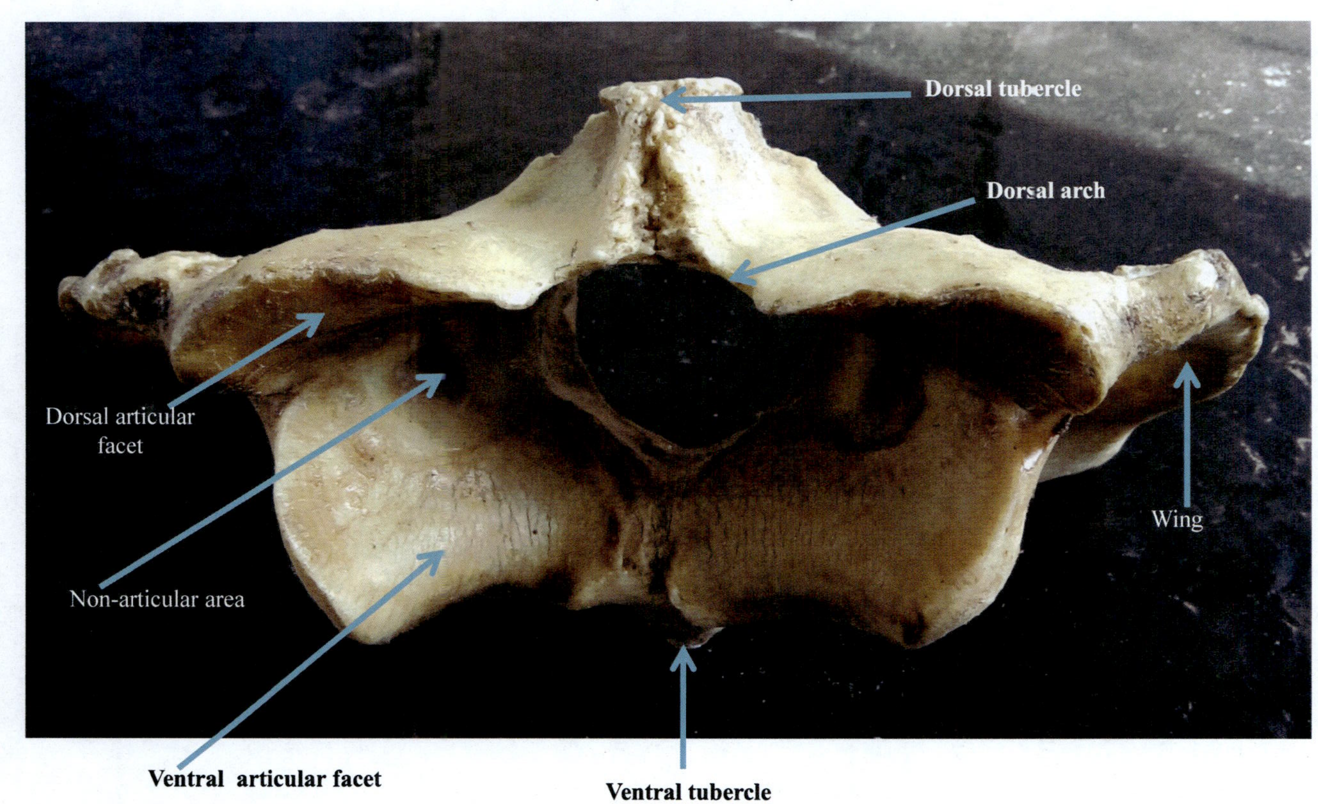

The Atlas

- The **atlas, or first cervical vertebra**, is uniquely structured, lacking both a body and spinous processes.
- It assumes a ring-like form, characterized by two laterally projecting curved plates known as the **wings**, which correspond to the transverse processes of other vertebrae.
- The dorsal aspect of the atlas features a transversely flattened articular surface, the fovea dentis, located caudally for articulation with the dens of the axis (the second cervical vertebra).
- Cranial to this surface lies a roughened area that serves as the attachment site for the ligamentum dentis, also known as the **odontoid ligament**.

Atlas (Ventro-lateral view)

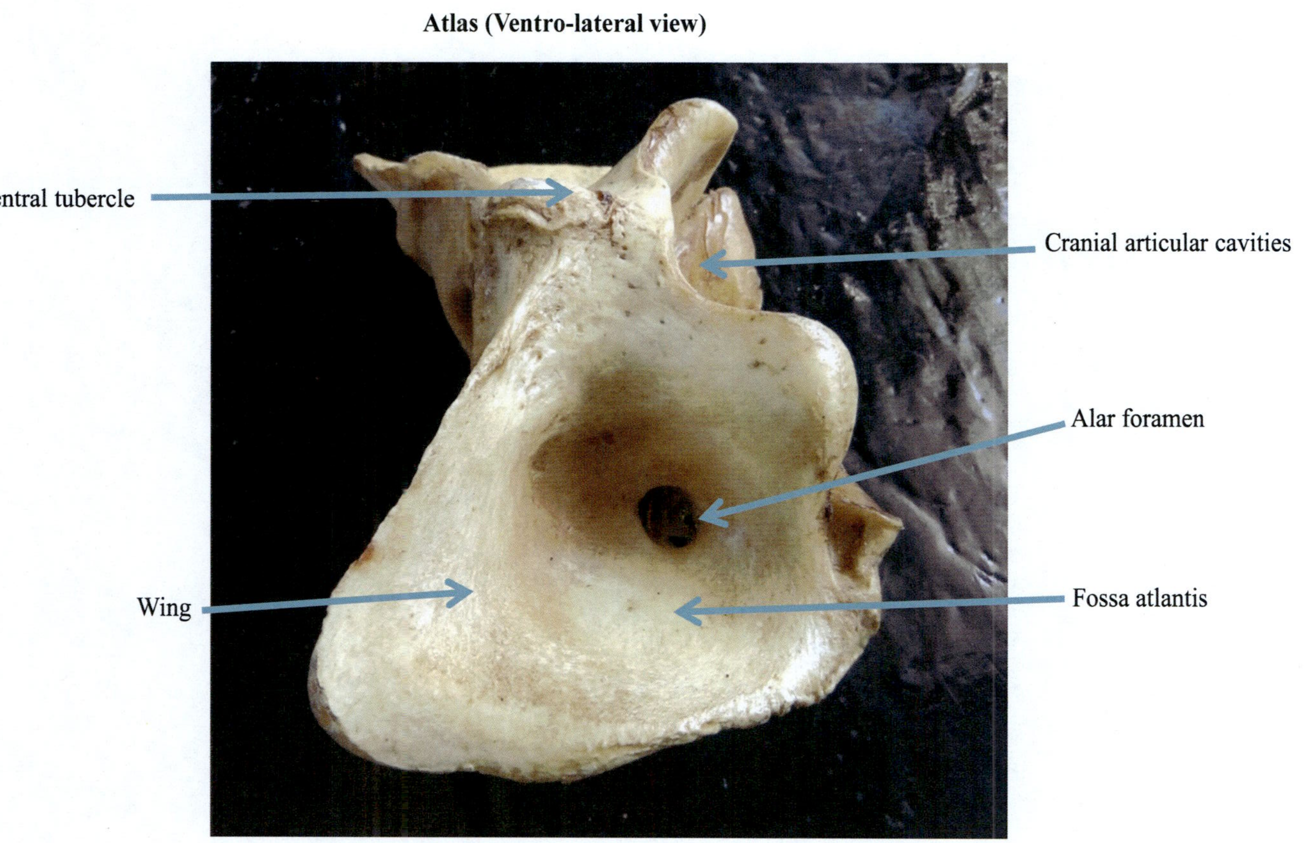

The Atlas

- The **omotransversarius muscle** derives its name from its insertion on the transverse process of the atlas (C1).
- The first cervical vertebra articulates with the occipital condyles, forming a synovial joint known as the **atlanto-occipital joint**.
- This joint facilitates the movement of the head, allowing for flexion and extension, or rocking motion, as the head tilts upward and downward.
- The space between the atlas and the occipital bone is referred to as the atlanto-occipital space, which plays a crucial role in the biomechanics of cranial movement.

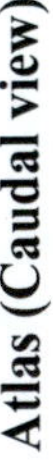
Atlas (Caudal view)
Caudal articular facet
Wing
Vertebral foramen
Fovea dentis
Ventral tubercle
Caudal articular facet
Wing

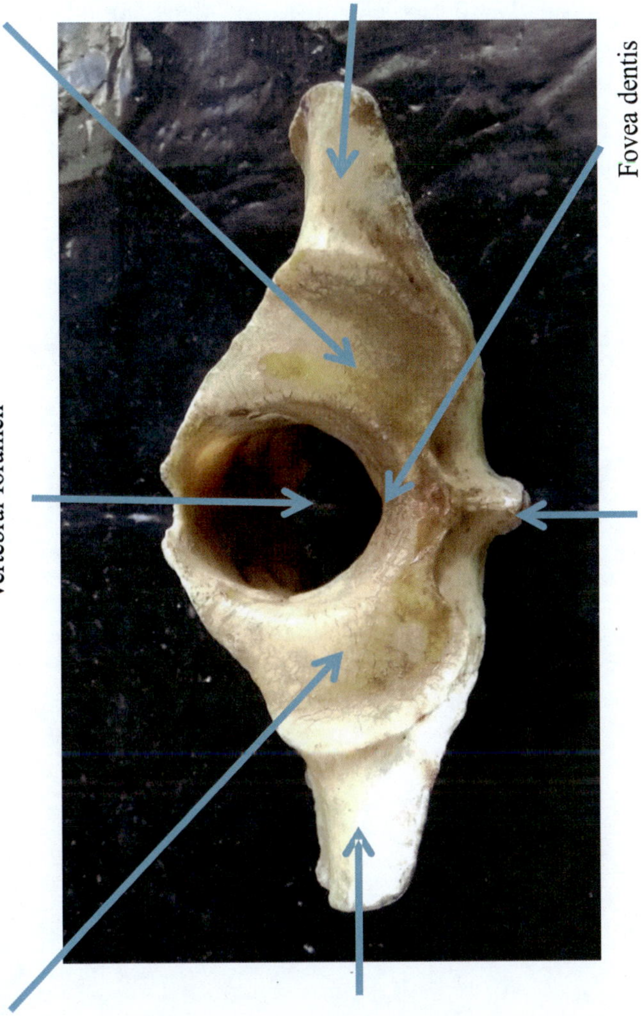

The Axis

- The **axis, or second cervical vertebra**, is characterized by its prominent spinous process, which is both elongated and broad when viewed from a lateral perspective.
- Additionally, the axis features the dens, or odontoid process, which extends cranially.
- Developmentally, the dens is considered a component of the atlas, or first cervical vertebra.
- It is the **longest of the vertebrae**. It features an odontoid process, which is characterized by its **spout-like shape**, broad dimensions, and a convex articular surface on its inferior aspect.

Axis (Caudodorsal View)

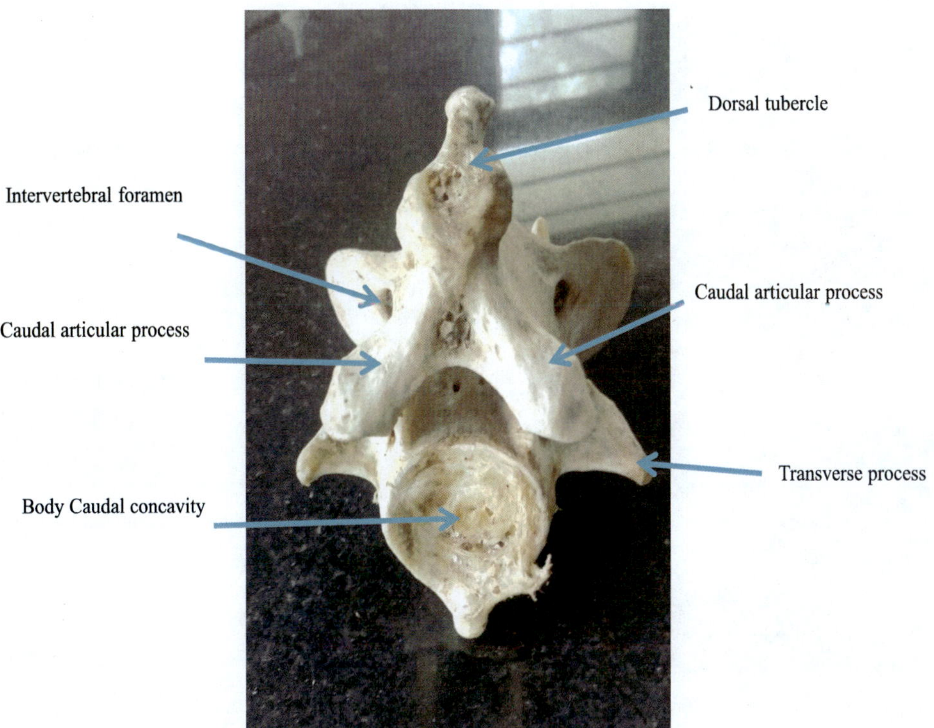

- The **cranial articular processes** are notably absent, while the caudal pair closely resembles those of the subsequent vertebrae.
- The **transverse processes** are small and undivided, projecting posteriorly. When present, the foramen transversarium manifests as an osseous canal traversing the root of the transverse process, characterized by anterior and posterior openings.
- The spinous process is large and robust, with a narrow summit cranially that thickens and widens caudally, providing attachment for the lamellar portion of the ligamentum nuchae and associated musculature.
- The **ventral spine** presents as a pronounced ridge, which becomes tuberculate at its posterior extremity.

Axis (Craniodorsal View)

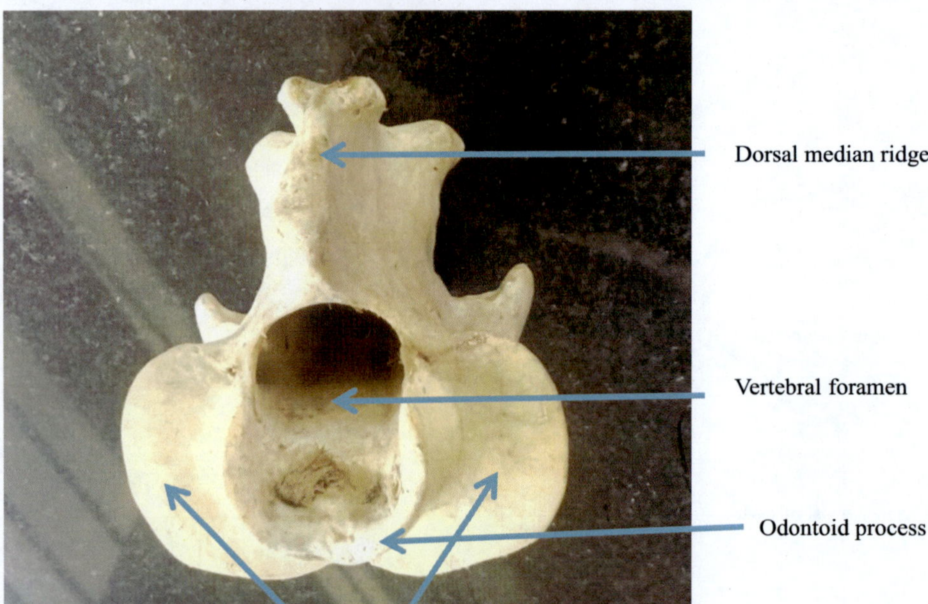

Nuchal ligament

- Cattle possess a specialized connective tissue support structure known as the nuchal ligament, which plays a critical role in accommodating their heavy heads while allowing for the flexibility required for grazing.
- This ligament provides essential support, reducing the muscular effort needed to elevate the head after foraging.
- When the head is lowered, the elastic nature of the nuchal ligament enables it to stretch and store energy, which can then assist in lifting the head back up, thereby facilitating efficient movement and feeding behaviors.

Axis (Ventro-lateral View)

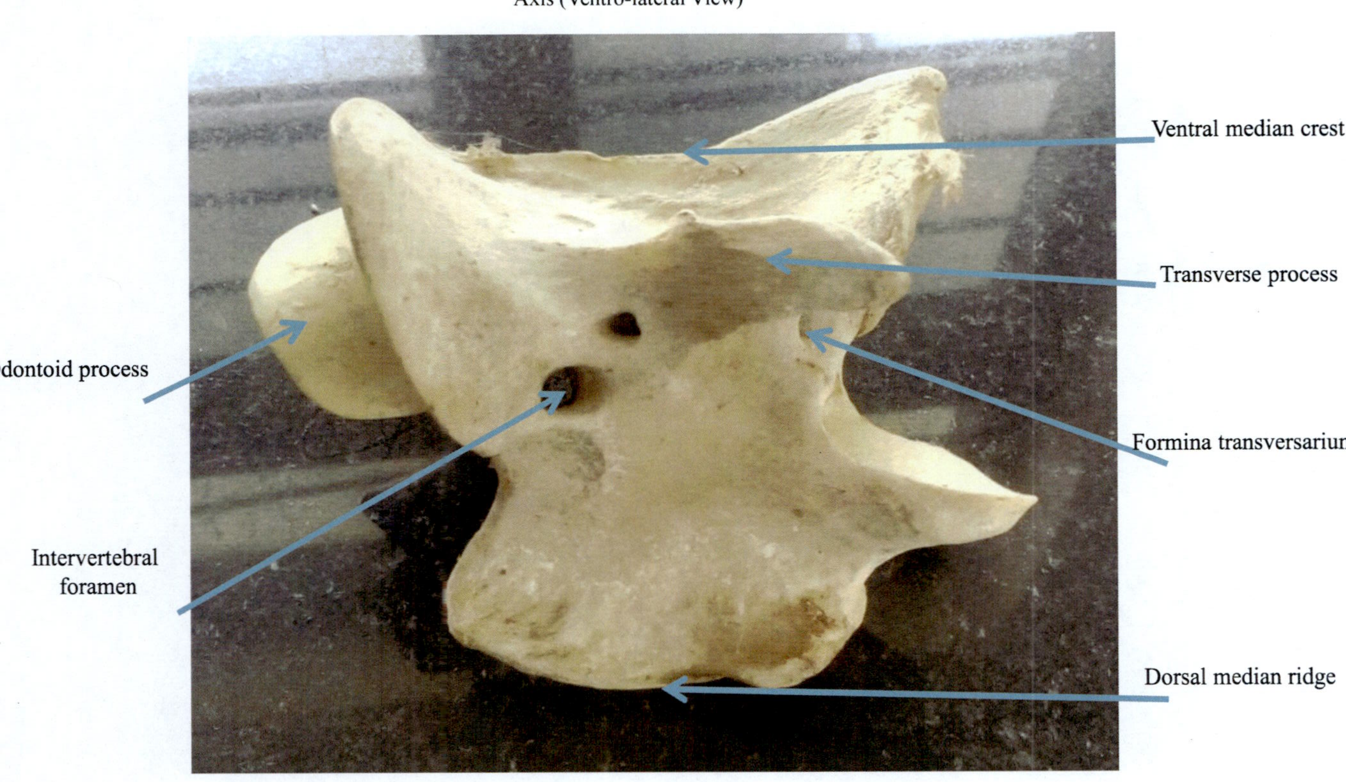

Funicular part and the laminar parts of Nuchal ligament

- The nuchal ligament in cattle is a paired structure comprising two distinct parts: the funicular part and the laminar part.
- The **funicular part** is located dorsally and extends from the occipital bone of the skull to the spinous processes of the first few thoracic vertebrae. It is elastic in nature and is continuous with the supraspinous ligament of the vertebral column.
- The **laminar part**, in contrast, has a sheet-like configuration and occupies the space between the funicular part and the cervical vertebrae. This portion serves to provide additional support and stability to the cervical region.

Axis (Ventral View)

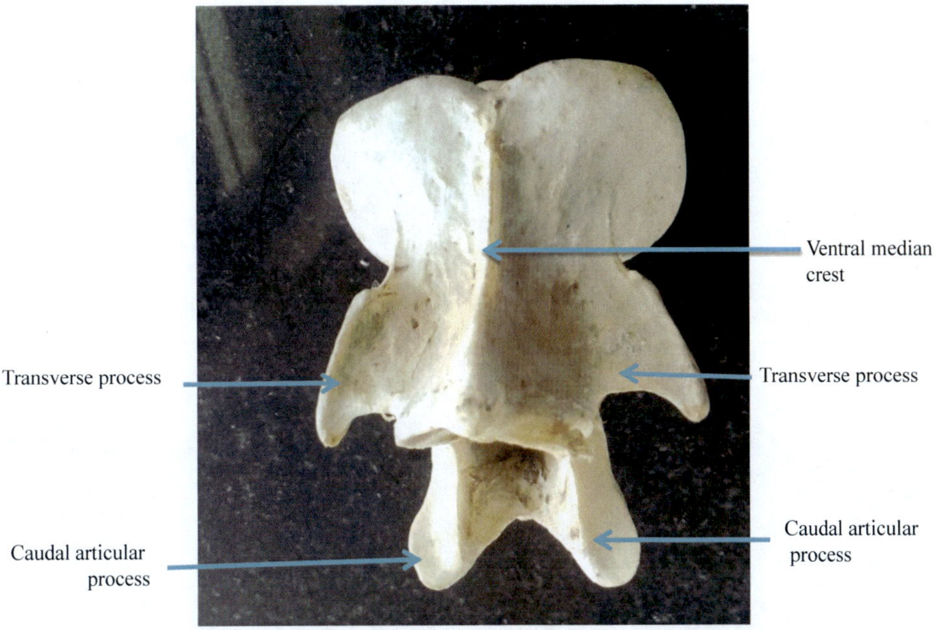

- **Bursae** can form in areas where the nuchal ligament is close to bone.
- **The cranial nuchal bursa** is located between the nuchal ligament and the dorsal arch of the atlas, while the caudal nuchal bursa is found between the ligament and the spinous process of the axis.
- **The supraspinous bursa** is situated between the supraspinous ligament and the prominent thoracic spinous processes (the withers).
- **Poll evil:** Infections of these bursae can lead to bursitis, with "poll evil" referring to cranial nuchal bursitis and "fistulous withers" indicating supraspinous bursitis. Notably, Brucella can cause fistulous withers, necessitating caution and culture of samples for diagnosis.

Axis (Cranio-dorsal View)

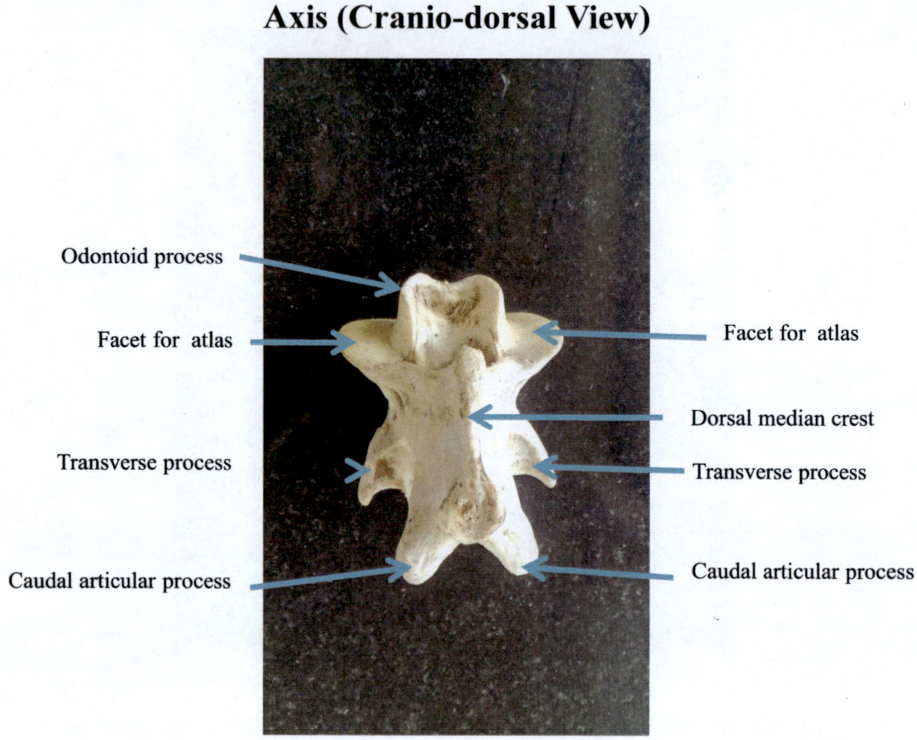

3rd to the 7th Vertebrae

- The vertebrae in this region have long bodies that decrease in length from the 3rd to the 7th.
- The ventral surface has a median spinous process that becomes less prominent caudally.
- The dorsal surface is flat for ligament attachment, and the ends of the vertebral bodies are concave and convex.
- The articular processes are large, and a continuous bone plate connects the cranial and caudal processes on each side.
- The transverse processes have a foramen (except in the 7th vertebra) for the passage of vessels and nerves.
- Each transverse process splits into upper and lower parts for muscle attachment. The spinous processes are thick, directed upwards and forwards, and increase in height from the 3rd to the 5th, with the 3rd often being bifid.

Typical Cervical Vertebra (Cranial View)

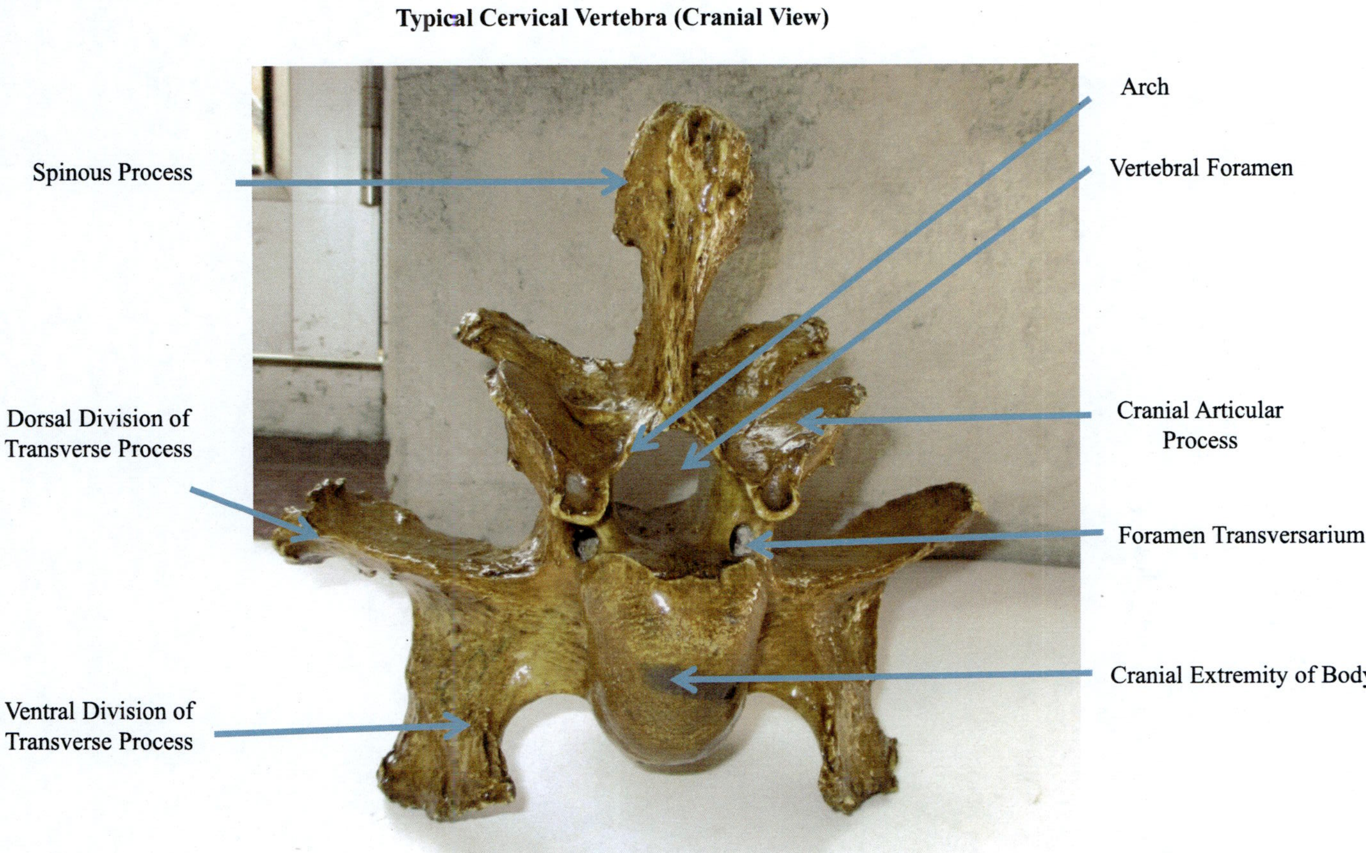

Diseases of the cervical spine

- Diseases of the cervical spine that involve the spinal cord are relatively uncommon in cattle but can present with significant neurological signs. Common conditions affecting the cervical spine include abscesses, osteomyelitis, and discospondylitis, all of which may result in generalized ataxia, proprioceptive deficits in the forelimbs, and tetraparesis.
- Cattle affected by discospondylitis may also exhibit marked stiffness of the neck.
- Other potential causes of cervical spine and spinal cord disorders in cattle include trauma, neoplasia, hypodermosis, and degenerative changes.
- Notably, animals with cervical spine or spinal cord lesions typically maintain normal demeanour, mental status, and cranial nerve function.

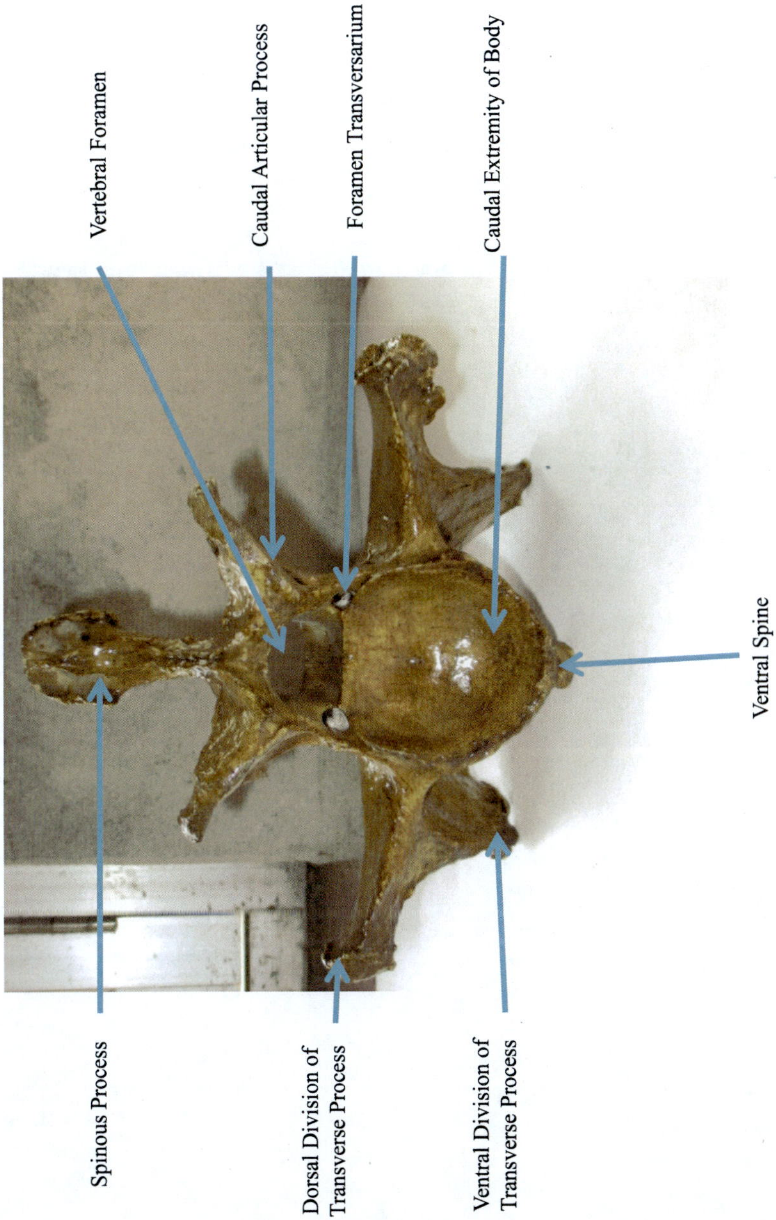

Typical Cervical Vertebra
(Caudal View)

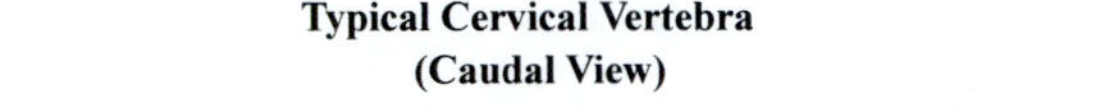

The sixth cervical vertebra

- The sixth cervical vertebra in cattle exhibits several distinctive features.
- The vertebral body is comparatively shorter and wider.
- The lower portion of the transverse process is more developed, plate-like in shape, and extends notably below and posteriorly relative to the body.
- The dorsal spine is longer than that of the fifth cervical vertebra. Notably, the ventral spine is absent.

6th Cervical Vertebra (Caudal View)

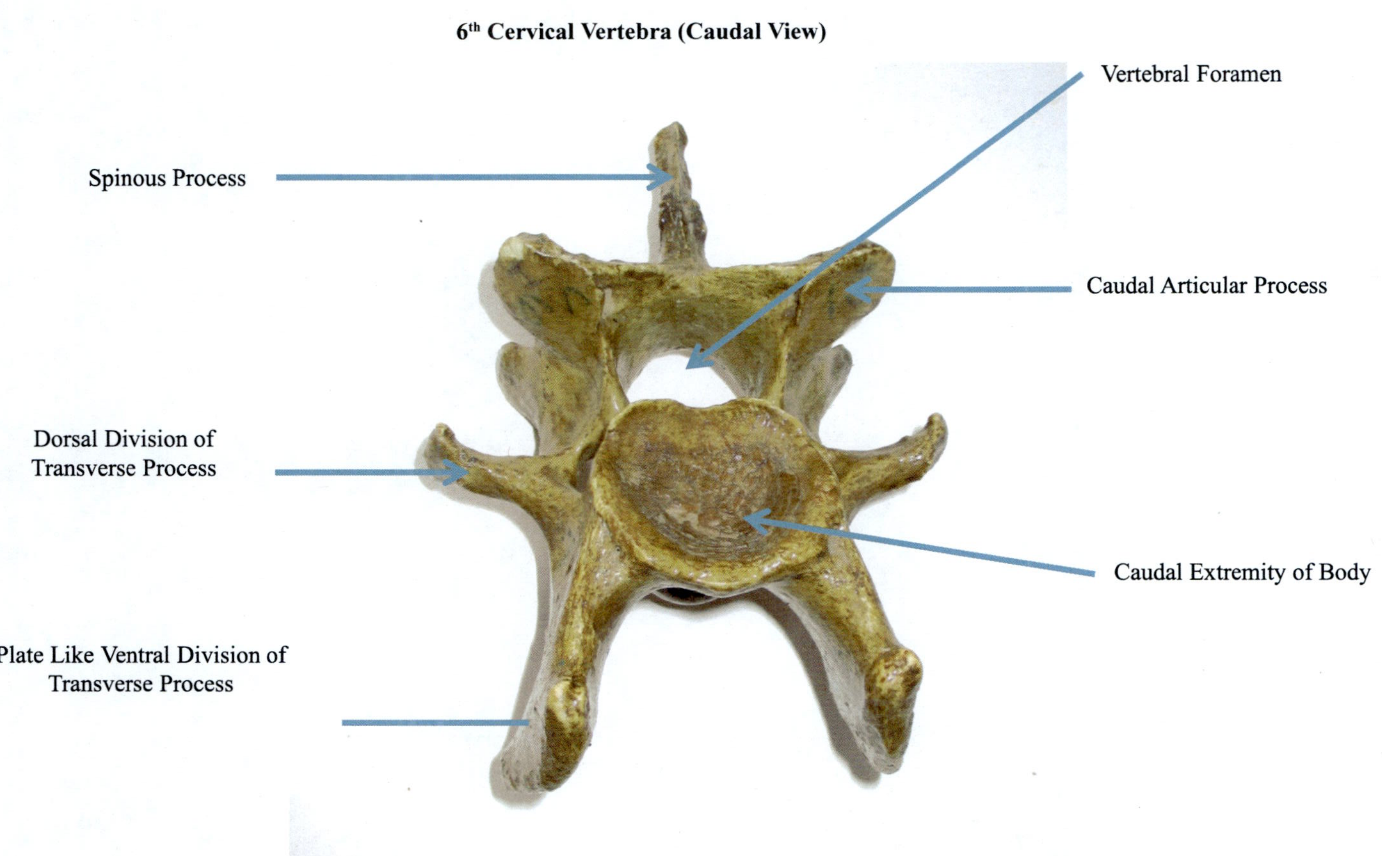

The jugular groove in cattle

- The jugular groove in cattle is a prominent anatomical feature along the neck, formed by the sternomandibularis (ventral) and cleidocephalicus (dorsal) muscles.
- It contains the jugular vein, which is large and superficial, making it easily accessible for blood collection, intravenous injections, and other veterinary procedures.
- The jugular vein in cattle plays an essential role in the circulation system, returning blood from the head, neck, and upper body to the heart.
- It carries deoxygenated blood from the head and neck back to the heart via the cranial vena cava.

6th Cervical Vertebra (Cranial View)

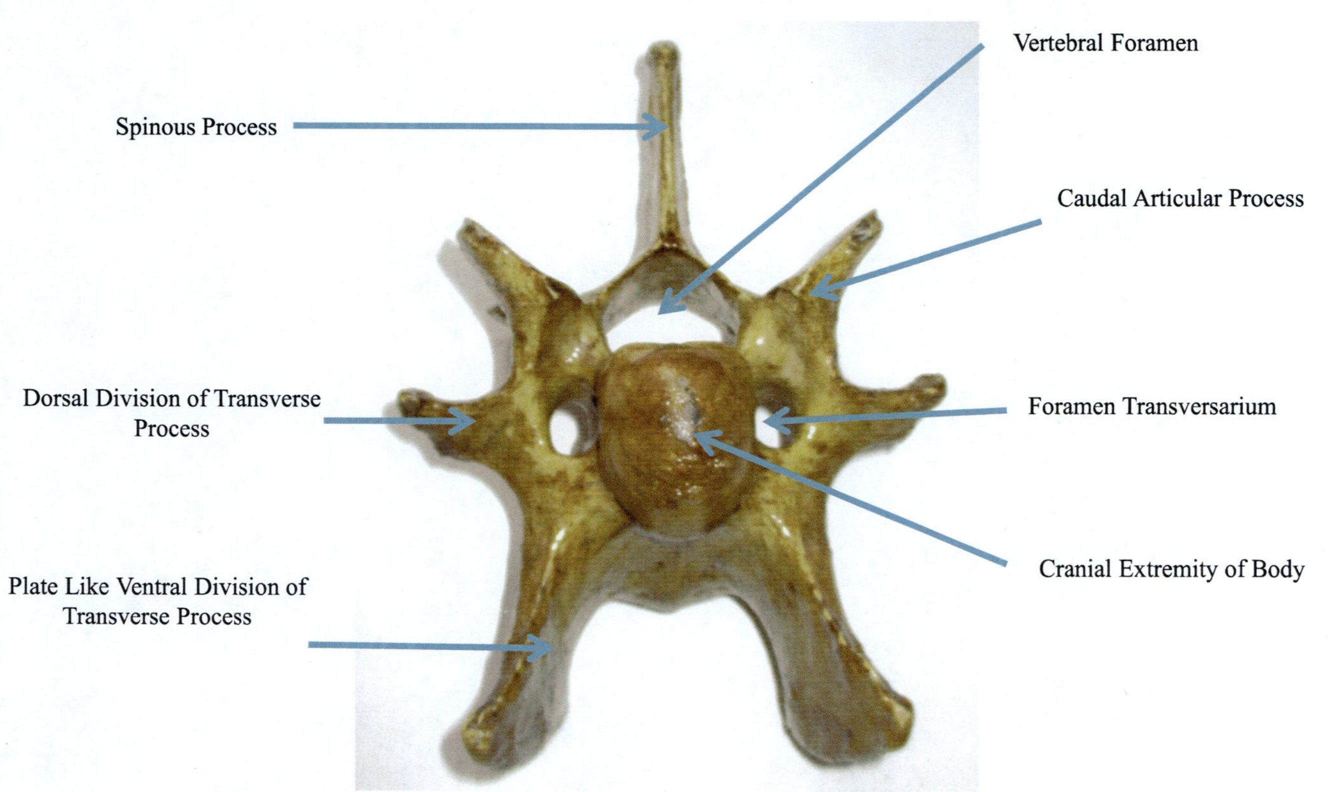

The vagus sympathetic trunk in cattle

- The vagus sympathetic trunk in cattle, like in other mammals, refers to a combination of the vagus nerve (cranial nerve X) and sympathetic fibers, which are involved in autonomic regulation, including control over heart rate, digestion, and respiratory function.
- The vagus nerve and sympathetic nervous system are components of the autonomic nervous system, which operates largely below the level of consciousness to regulate various bodily functions.
- Damage to the vagus nerve can impair the parasympathetic control of the gastrointestinal system, leading to conditions like vagus indigestion, which is a common problem in cattle that affects their ability to process food properly.

6th Cervical Vertebra (Antero-ventral View)

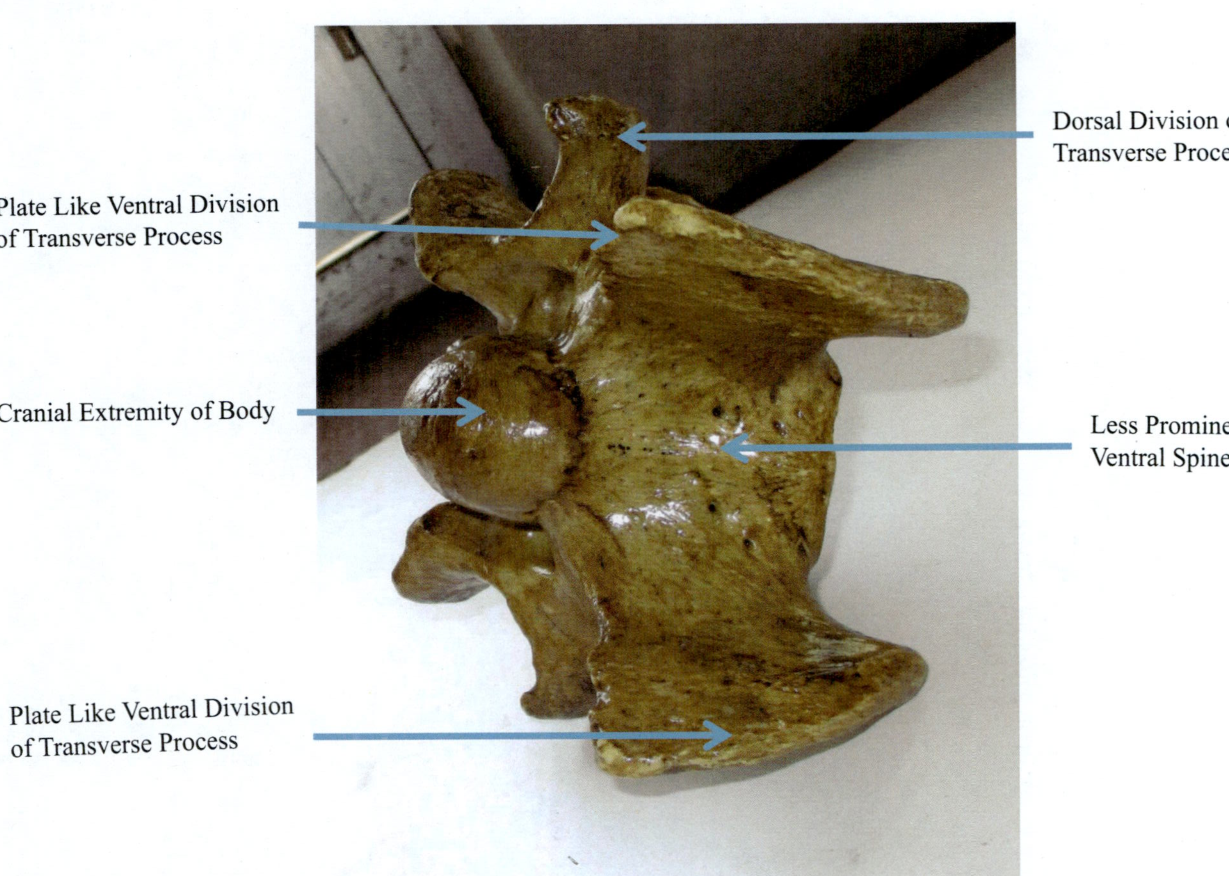

The Seventh Cervical Vertebra

The seventh cervical vertebra in cattle, known as the vertebra prominens, is distinguished by several unique features:

1. **Short body**: It is the shortest among the cervical vertebrae.
2. **Single transverse process**: Unlike the others, its transverse process is undivided and lacks the foramen transversarium.
3. **Well-developed spinous process**: The spinous process is prominent and gently inclines forward, forming a notable plate of bone.
4. **Costal facets**: It has concave costal facets at the posterior end of the body that, with the first dorsal vertebra, form a cup-shaped cavity for the first rib's head.
5. **Absence of ventral spine**: Unlike other vertebrae, it does not have a ventral spine.

7th Cervical Vertebra (Caudal View)

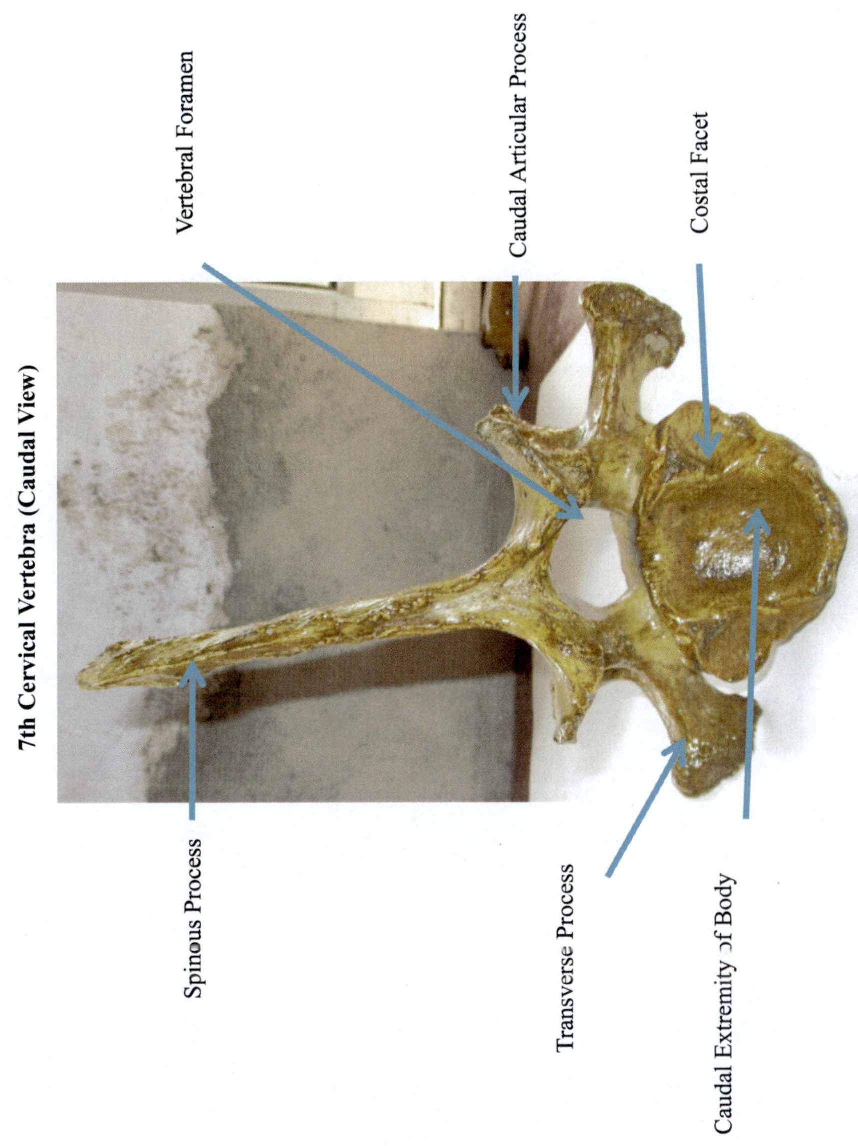

Diskospondylitis in cattle

- Diskospondylitis in cattle is mainly caused by bacterial infections, although fungal infections can also play a role.
- Common bacterial pathogens include Trueperella pyogenes, Staphylococcus aureus, Escherichia coli, Brucella abortus, and Actinomyces species.
- Fungal infections, such as Aspergillus or Histoplasma, are rare causes.
- The infection typically spreads to the intervertebral discs and vertebral bodies via the bloodstream (hematogenous spread) from other infected body parts or through direct extension from nearby tissues or skin. Trauma, such as fractures or surgery, can also increase the risk of infection.

7th Cervical Vertebra (Cranial View)

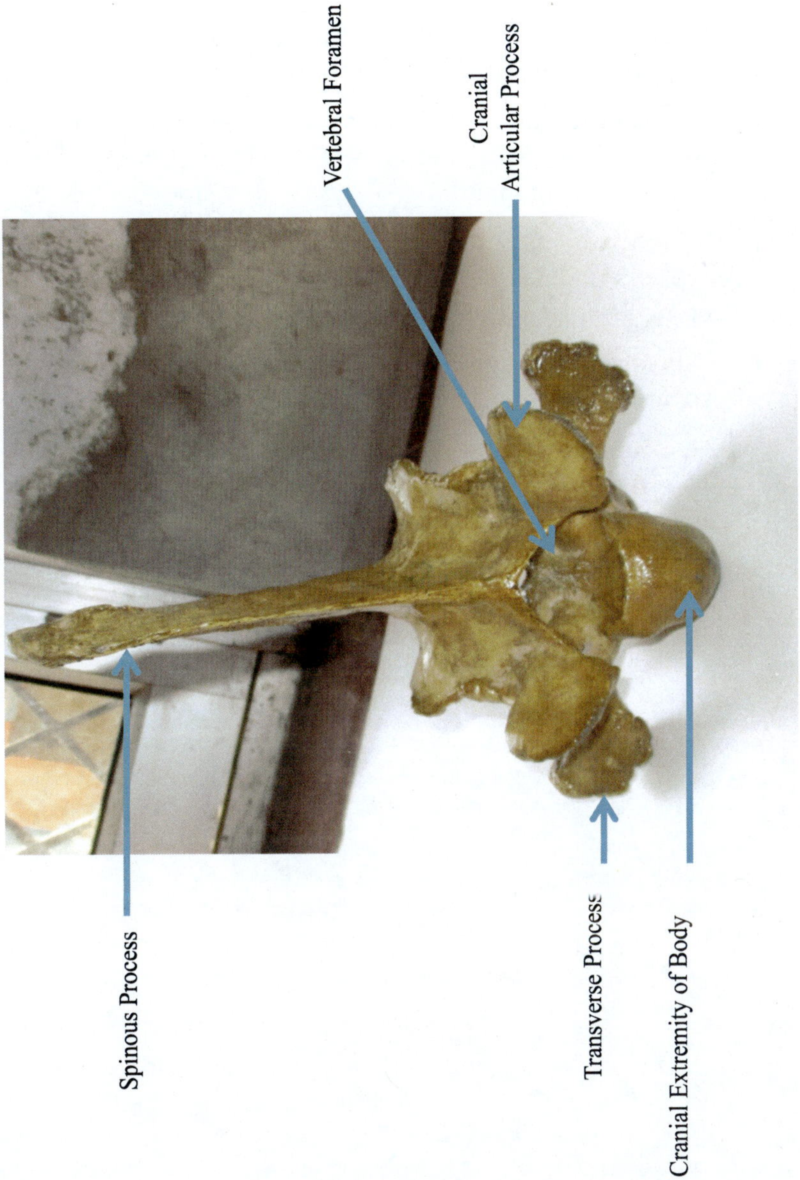

Vertebral Foramen

Cranial
Articular Process

Spinous Process

Transverse Process

Cranial Extremity of Body

Diskospondylitis

- **Diskospondylitis** in cattle is a rare, but serious, condition that affects the intervertebral discs and adjacent vertebrae of the spine.
- It is characterized by inflammation and infection of the intervertebral discs (the soft tissue between the vertebrae), and the adjacent bony structures of the spine.
- Diskospondylitis is a potentially debilitating condition (severe pain, lameness, and neurological dysfunction) in cattle that can lead to severe consequences if left untreated.
- Early diagnosis, appropriate antimicrobial treatment, and supportive care are critical to achieving a favorable outcome.
- Close monitoring and veterinary intervention are necessary to manage this condition effectively.

The carotid artery in cattle

- The carotid artery in cattle is a major blood vessel that supplies blood to the head and neck. It is a crucial part of the circulatory system in bovines, as it provides oxygenated blood to the brain, face, and neck structures.
- The carotid artery in cattle is located in the neck region and can be found running along the ventral (lower) part of the neck, just beneath the trachea (windpipe) and slightly to the side of the esophagus.
- It runs deeper than the jugular vein, which is also found in the same region.

Thoracic Vertebra

- 13 in numbers
- Costal facet on the body
- Facet for tubercle of rib on transverse process
- Large, narrow spinous process slopes upward and backward.
- **1st Thoracic Vertebra**

a) Wide and dorso-ventrally flattened body

b) Much larger articular processes than those of other thoracic vertebrae

- Distinct mammillary process on Last 3 or 4
- Absence of the Caudal pair of costal facets distinguished the last thoracic vertebra

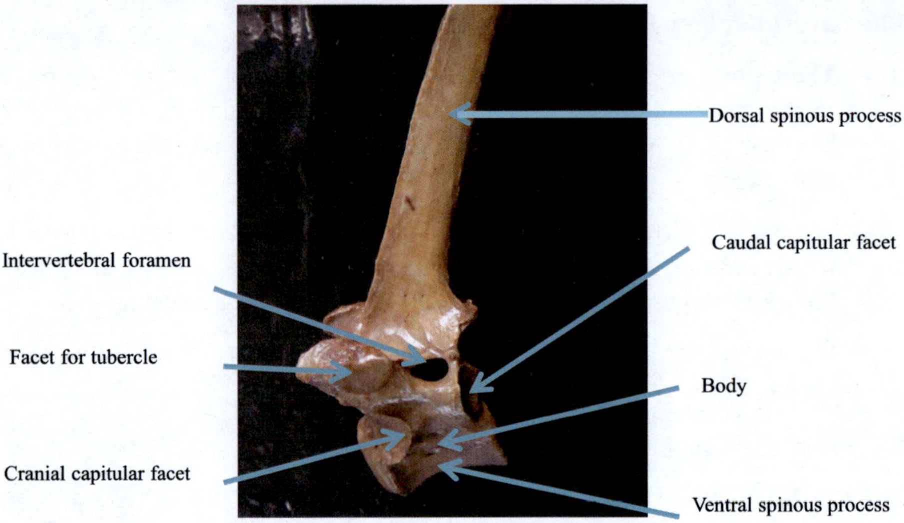

Dorsal spinous process
Caudal capitular facet
Intervertebral foramen
Facet for tubercle
Body
Cranial capitular facet
Ventral spinous process

Thoracic vertebrae of cattle

- The spinous processes of the thoracic vertebrae exhibit notable characteristics throughout the spinal column.
- The first spinous process is significantly elevated, while the second and third are typically the most prominent.
- As one moves caudally, there is a gradual decrease in the height of these processes. Initially, the caudal slope is slight, but it becomes more pronounced by the tenth vertebra.
- The last spinous process is vertical in orientation and resembles lumbar characteristics. The apex of the first spinous process is usually pointed, while those located further caudad display a noticeable thickening.
- Additionally, the width of the spinous processes generally narrows from the fifth to the eleventh vertebra.
- While both lateral borders of the spinous processes are typically thin and sharp, the last three or four processes may exhibit thicker caudal margins.

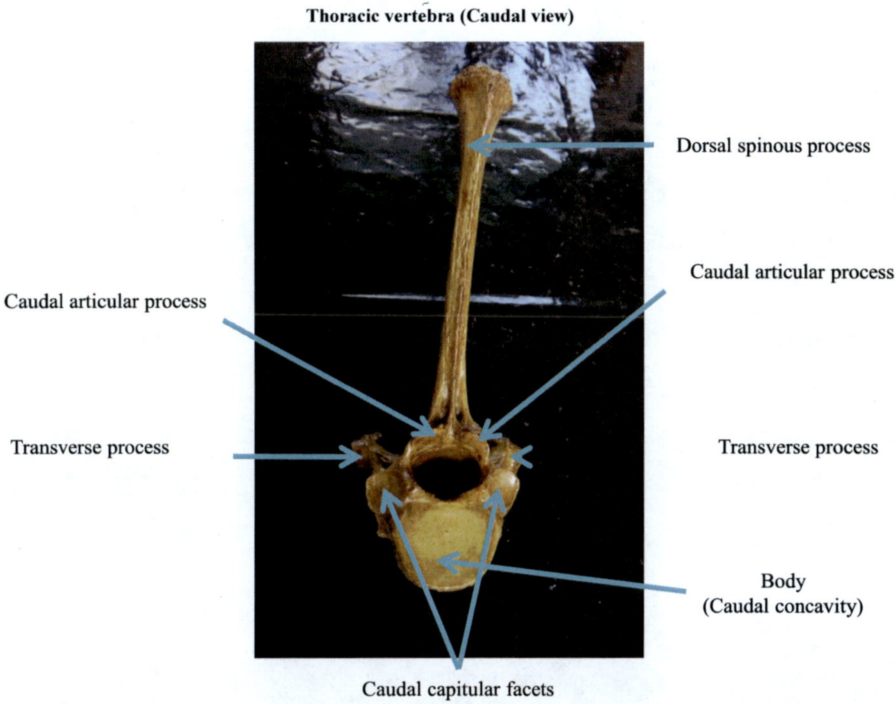

- At the **caudal edge** of each thoracic vertebra, one can observe a notch located at the base of the vertebral arch, just dorsal to the vertebral body.
- This notch serves as the foundation for either an intervertebral foramen or a lateral vertebral foramen.
- When the notch is closed, it results in the formation of a lateral vertebral foramen; conversely, if the notch remains open, it gives rise to an intervertebral foramen.
- The **spinal nerve** that traverses either of these foramina will subsequently course laterally along the caudal edge of the adjacent rib.

Thoracic vertebra (Cranio-lateral view)

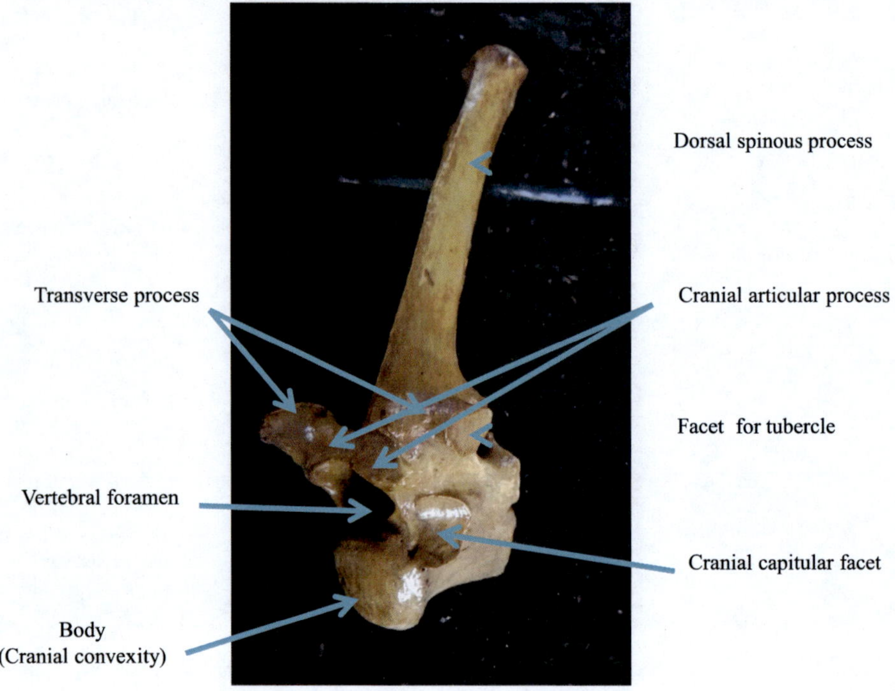

- In cattle, the **thoracic spinal cord segments**, along with the first two lumbar segments, are positioned caudally, aligning closely with the intervertebral discs.
- The epaxial muscle system in cattle is located dorsally to the transverse processes of the vertebrae, where it is closely associated with the vertebral column and ribs.
- This system is organized into three main muscle groups, arranged from lateral to medial: the iliocostalis, longissimus, and transversospinalis.

Lumbar Vertebra

- 6 in number
- Characterized by the size and form of their transverse processes
- Mammillary processes fused with the Cranial articular processes
- The transverse processes project outward and usually curve slightly downward
- The length of transverse processes increases to the third or fourth, and then diminishes to the last, which is the shortest

The Lumbar Vertebrae

- The lumbar vertebrae are distinct from the thoracic vertebrae in several key features.
- Notably, the bodies of the lumbar vertebrae are longer and more uniform in shape.
- Additional regional characteristics include the absence of costal facets, a shorter height and more forward-sloping spinous processes, and long, flattened transverse processes that project laterally.
- The articular processes are interlocking, and the lumbar vertebrae often feature prominent mammillary processes, with accessory processes occasionally present as well.

Lumbar vertebra (Craniodorsal view)

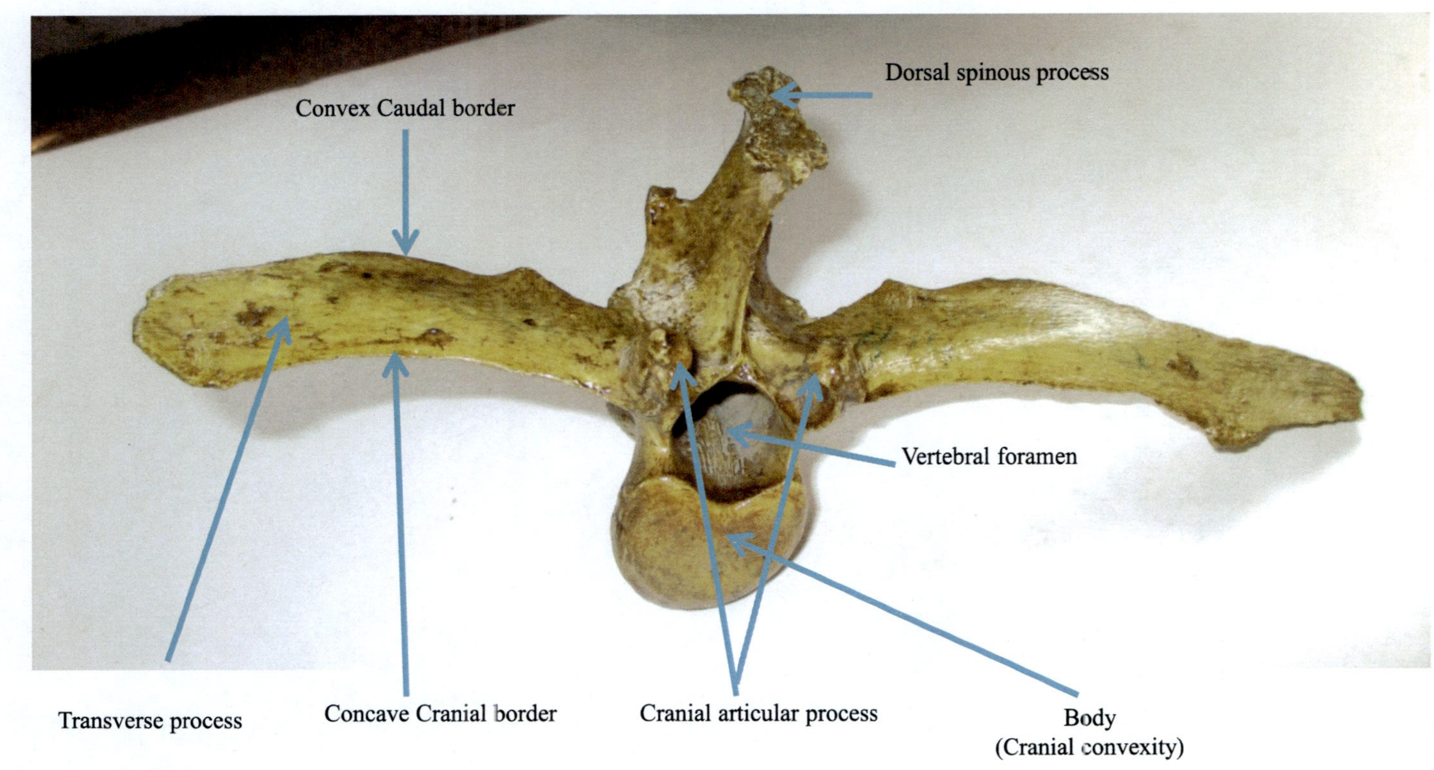

The paralumbar fossa

- The paralumbar fossa is a depression located in the upper flank region of the cow, specifically ventral to the transverse processes of the lumbar vertebrae.
- It can be most clearly observed in a live animal, providing a natural indentation that is clinically significant in veterinary procedures.
- The fossa is important in surgical and anesthetic practices because it serves as an entry point for various procedures. For instance: Rumen cannulation, foreign body removal and Cecal access etc.

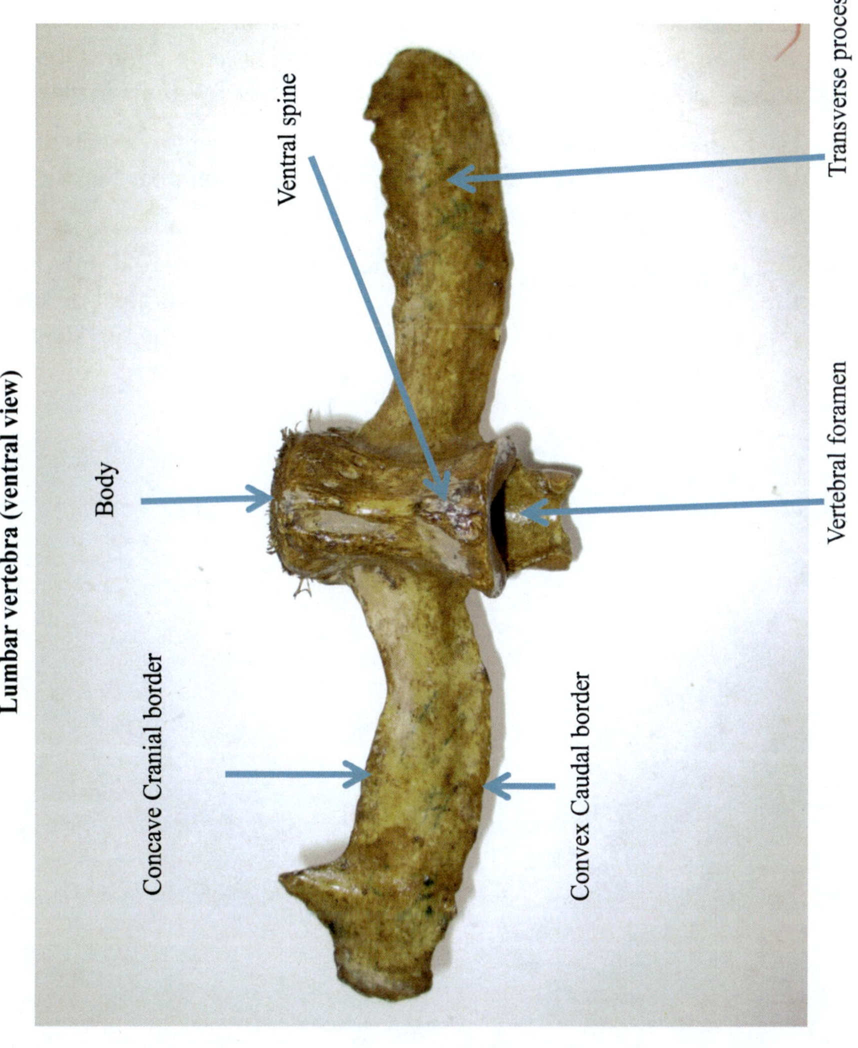
Lumbar vertebra (ventral view)
Body
Concave Cranial border
Ventral spine
Transverse process
Vertebral foramen
Convex Caudal border

- **Rumen cannulation:** This is a common procedure where the left paralumbar fossa is incised to access the rumen. A fistula is inserted, allowing for long-term access to the rumen for sampling or monitoring, often used in research or for managing certain conditions in cattle.
- **Foreign body removal:** In cases where a foreign object has been ingested and is lodged in the rumen, the left paralumbar fossa provides an approach for its removal.
- The paralumbar fossa, located on the right side of the abdomen, is used for cecal access in cases like cecal dilation or other surgical procedures. It is also an important landmark for veterinarians during physical exams and when making precise incisions for various procedures

Lumbar vertebra (Caudodorsal view)

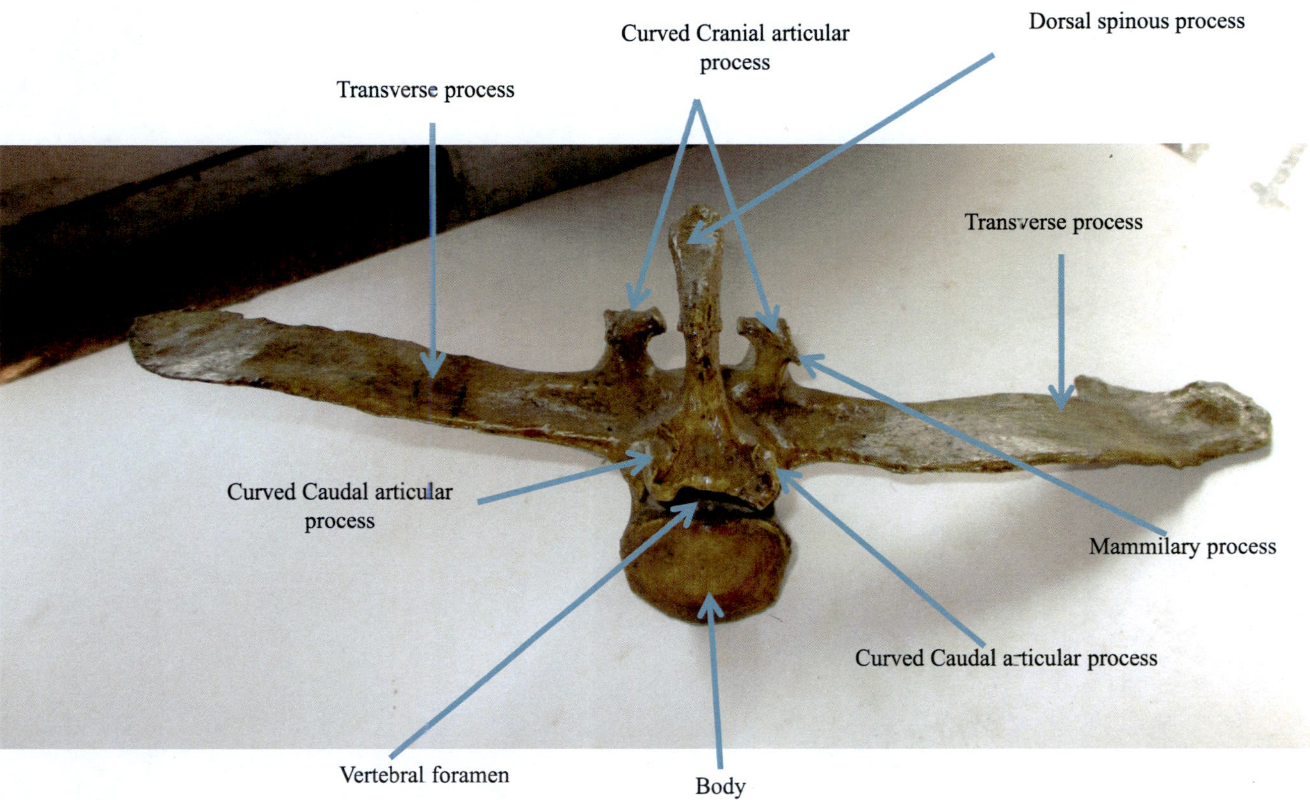

- **Hardware Disease** (Traumatic Reticuloperitonitis) occurs when sharp foreign objects, such as nails or wire, are ingested by cows and end up in the reticulum, the cranial part of the ruminant stomach. The reticulum's honeycomb-like structure helps slow ingesta transit for nutrient absorption, but it also increases the risk of sharp objects puncturing the wall. When this happens, the object can cause peritonitis (inflammation of the abdominal lining), abscesses, and in severe cases, penetrate through the diaphragm to the pericardial sac around the heart, leading to pericarditis and pleuritis.
- To prevent this, a magnet is often placed in the reticulum to attract and hold metallic objects, stopping them from causing harm.

Muscles of the Sublumbar Region

The muscles of the sublumbar region are located deep within the ventral aspect of the lumbar vertebrae and the cranial surface of the ilium. These muscles not only occupy the sublumbar region but also extend both cranially and caudally, contributing to the formation of the roof of the abdominal cavity. They are in close proximity to the abdominal viscera. The key muscles of the sublumbar region include:

- Psoas minor
- Psoas major
- Iliacus
- Quadratus lumborum
- Intertransversarales lumborum

Sacrum

- **Formed by the fusion of five vertebrae**
    - 4 Dorsal Sacral Foramina
    - 4 Ventral Sacral Foramina
    - Median Sacral Crest (fusion of dorsal spinous process)
    - Lateral Sacral Crest (fusion of articular processes)
- **Base**
    a) Directed forward and relatively very wide
    b) Presents centrally the body of the first sacral segment
    c) The alae or wings is lateral parts of the base
- **Apex**
    a) The Caudal(Caudal) aspect of the last sacral vertebra
    b) Very small
    c) Triangular Caudal opening of the sacral canal

Sacrum (Dorsal view)

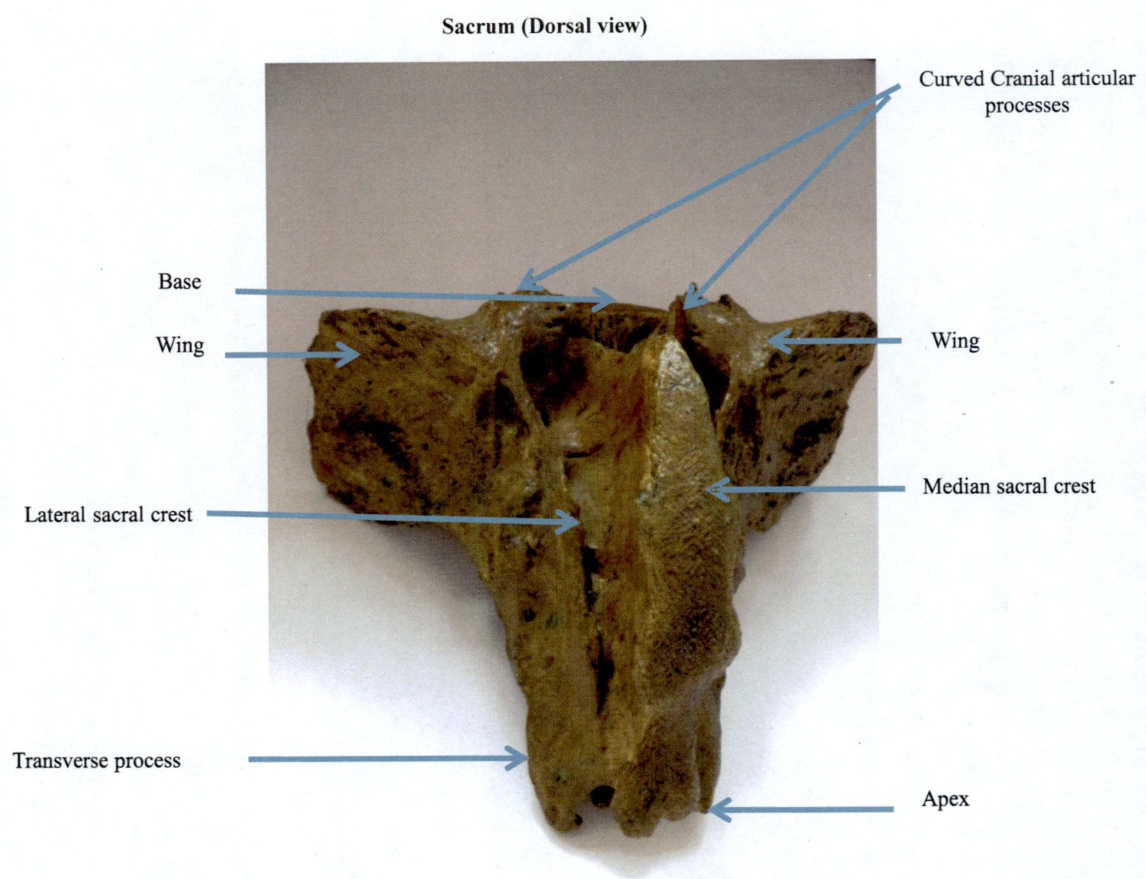

Sacrum

- **The pelvic surface** of the sacrum in cattle is concave both horizontally and vertically, marked by a central groove (sulcus vasculosus) that traces the path of the median sacral artery.
- The ventral sacral foramina are large. The wings of the sacrum curve ventrally and cranially; they are short, quadrangular, and compressed in the cranio-caudal direction, with a high dorsal-to-ventral height.
- The body of the first sacral segment is very wide, and the entrance to the sacral canal is correspondingly wide and low.
- The lateral borders of the sacrum are thin, sharp, and irregular. The caudal end of the medial crest forms a pointed projection over the opening of the sacral canal.

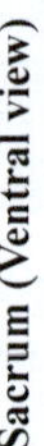

Sacrum (Ventral view)

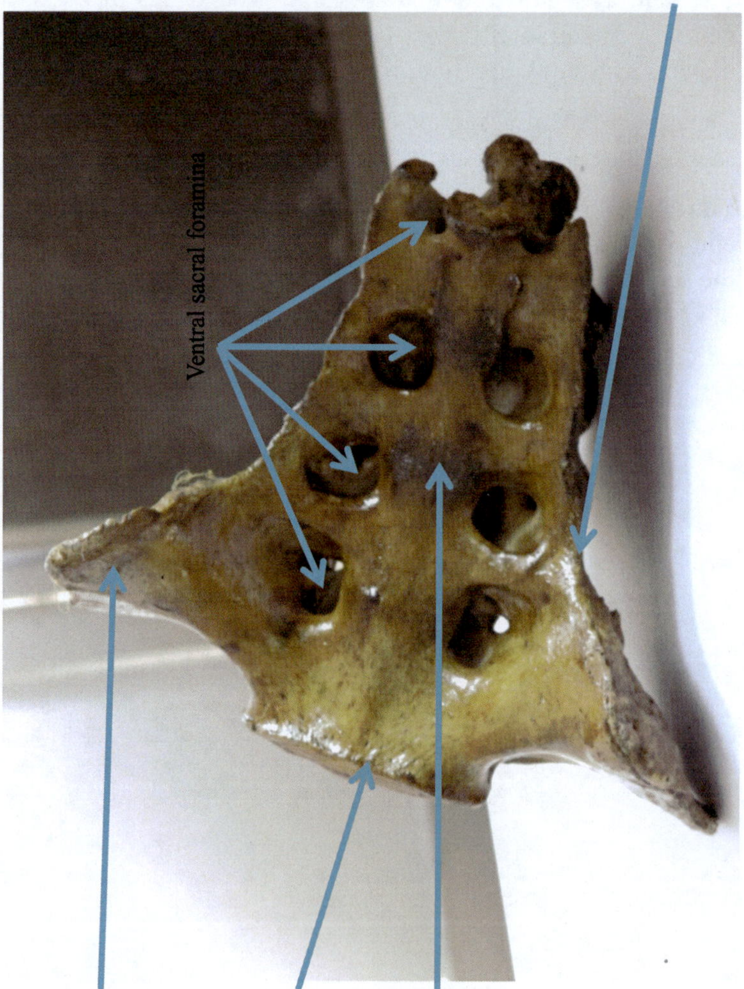

- **The sacral promontory:** It is an important anatomical feature in the context of the pelvis. Specifically, it refers to the cranial edge of the first sacral vertebra (S1) in mammals, including cattle. This prominence serves as a key landmark in the pelvic region.
- The sacrum is a critical anatomical structure in cattle that plays a key role in both locomotion and reproductive function.
- Abnormalities or injuries in the sacral region can lead to significant clinical problems, including lameness, birth complications, and overall decreased performance.

Sacrum (Craniodorsal view)

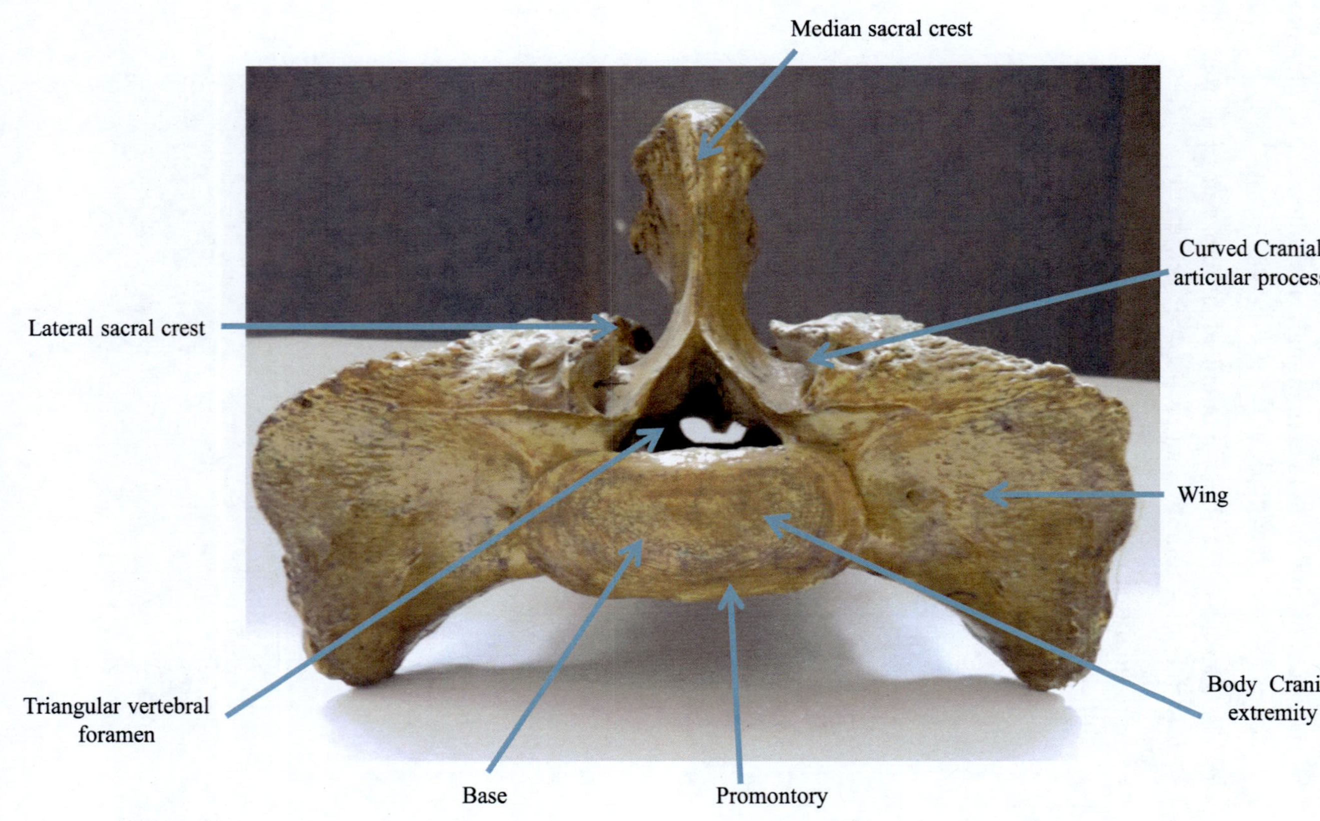

- **The sacrosciatic ligament:** It is a broad sheet of connective tissues that extends from the sacrum to the ilium and ischium, with slight variations between bovine and equine species.
- The caudal, thickened margin of this ligament is homologous to the sacrotuberous ligament found in dogs.
- Additionally, the sacrosciatic ligament contributes to the formation of the pelvic outlet's boundary.
- Indications of impending parturition in cows include the relaxation of the sacrosciatic ligament. As the cow approaches calving, the tail head lifts, and the sacrosciatic ligament becomes more relaxed, signaling the onset of labor.

Sacrum (Caudodorsal view)

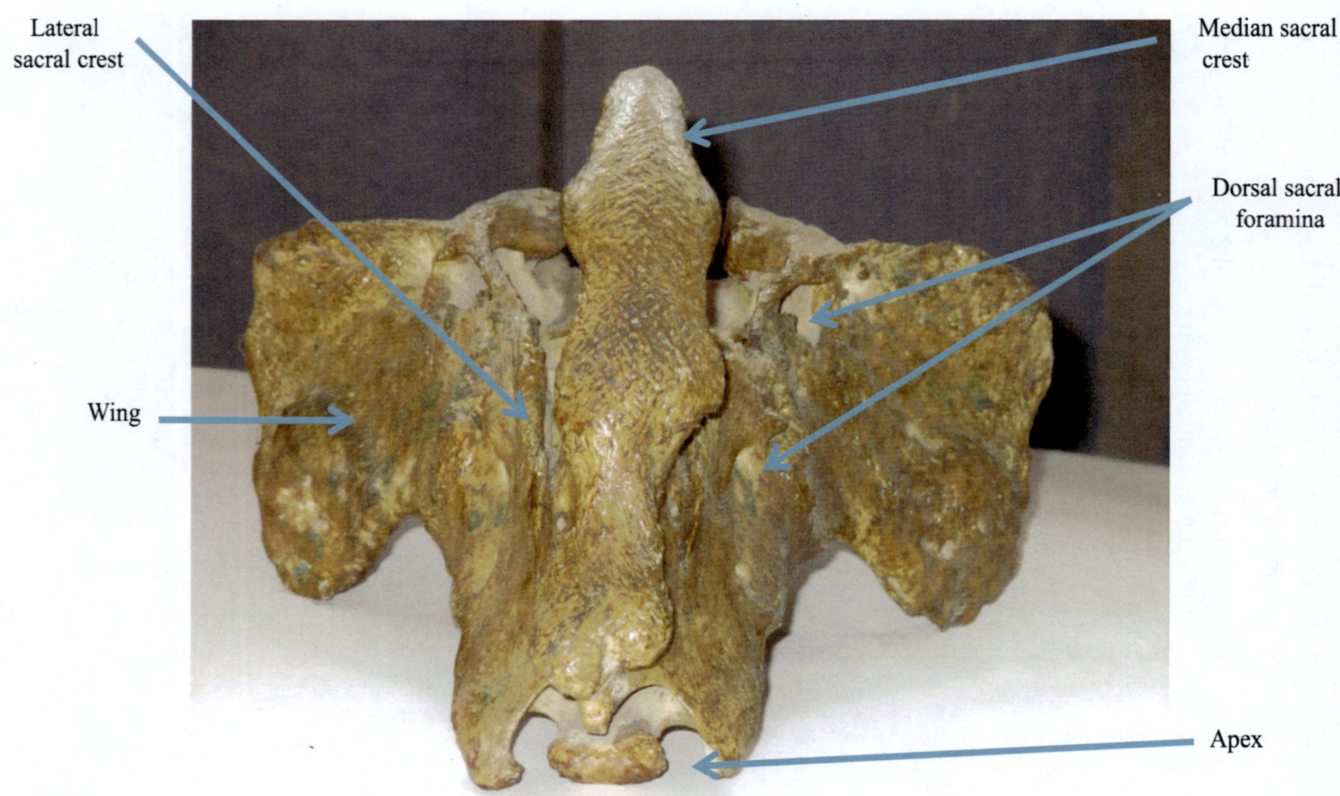

The sacral plexus in cattle

- The sacral plexus in cattle is a complex network of nerves located in the pelvic region, formed by the ventral branches of the sacral spinal nerves.
- It is a key structure in the peripheral nervous system, responsible for innervating muscles and skin of the pelvic limb and perineal area.
- The sacral plexus is involved in controlling movements of the hindlimbs and certain functions in the pelvic organs.
- The sacral plexus is typically formed from the ventral branches of the last lumbar (L6) and the first two sacral (S1, S2) spinal nerves.

Sciatic nerve and Pudendal nerve

- Sciatic nerve is the largest nerve arising from the sacral plexus. It supplies motor innervation to the muscles of the thigh and lower leg and sensory innervation to the skin of the hindlimb.
- Pudendal nerve is the nerve provides sensory and motor innervation to the perineal region, including the anus and external genitalia.
- In cattle, injuries to this area can occur during trauma, parturition (especially with dystocia), or as a result of certain diseases affecting the nervous system, like infections or nerve compression.

Coccygeal Vertebra

- Vary considerably in number
- From cranial to caudal series they become reduced in size and with the exception of a few at the beginning of the series, distally consist of bodies only
- Functional articular processes are not present but small rudiments of the Cranial pair commonly occur
- Relatively large plate like transverse processes project horizontally outward
- A pair of ventral spines (Haemal process) which form a groove (Sulcus vasculosus) for the middle coccygeal artery

Coccygeal Vertebra (Dorsal view)

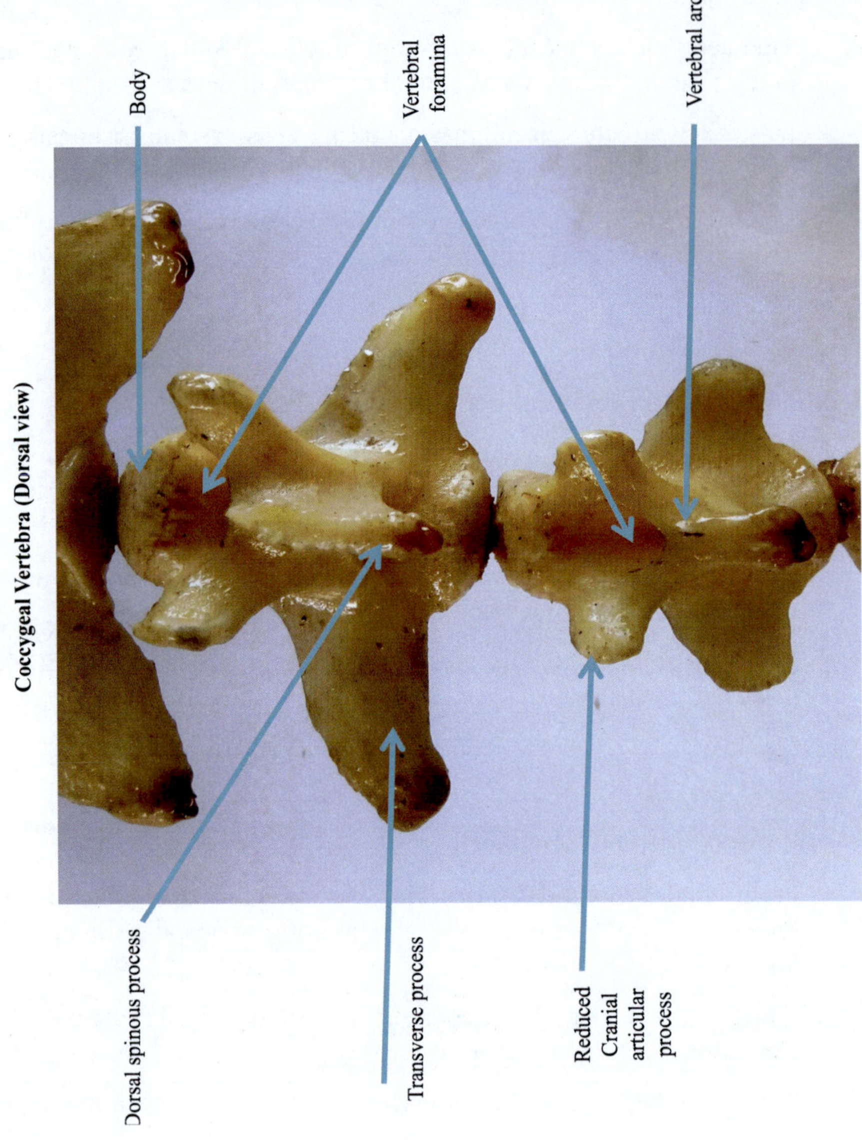

Median caudal (or "tail") vein

- In addition to the external jugular vein, the median caudal (or "tail") vein is another common site for blood collection in cattle. It is also used for recording of pulse in cattle.
- To access it, the tail should be raised, and the vein can be found in the proximal ventral third of the tail, between two adjacent tail vertebrae.
- Care must be taken to avoid the hemal arches of the caudal vertebrae in this area.

Coccygeal Vertebra (Ventral view)

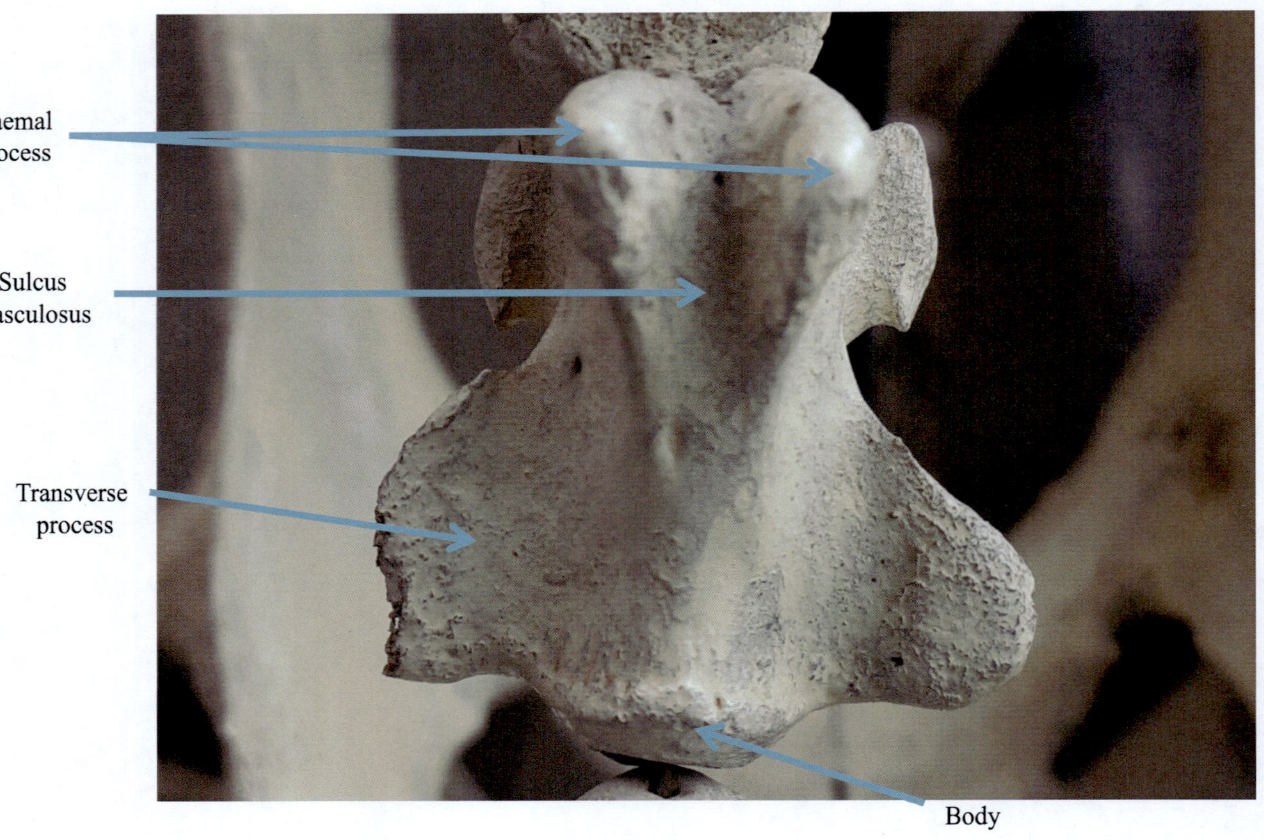

Epidural anesthesia in cattle

- Epidural anesthesia can be induced by accessing the epidural space at three potential interarcuate sites, depending on the area of interest: (i) L6–S1 (ii) S5–Cd1, and (iii) Cd1–Cd2.
- The most common sites for epidural administration in cattle, camels, and buffalos are the sacrococcygeal intervertebral space (S5-Cd1) and first intercoccygeal intervertebral space (Cd1-Cd2).
- Care should be taken during epidural puncture, as there is a risk of hemorrhage if the internal vertebral venous plexus is inadvertently punctured.

Clinical significance of tail

- Tail tone and movement are used to assess: spinal cord injuries, especially in the sacrococcygeal region, obstetric paralysis (e.g., following dystocia) and cauda equina syndrome.
- Tail injuries (e.g., fractures, dislocations, hematomas) can result from: rough handling (e.g., tail twisting), trauma (e.g., getting caught in machinery or gates) and tail docking complications (mainly in calves or show animals).
- Increased tail movement or lifting can be a sign of estrus in cows.
- Tail chalk or paint is also used in estrus detection systems in dairy farms.
- Tail flaccidity or tone can give clues to neurological status.

Ribs

- Sternal Ribs (8 pairs)
- Asternal Ribs (5 pairs)
- Shaft
- Angle

- **Two Extremities**

  a) Vertebral

  b) Sternal

- **Vertebral Extremity**

  a) Head

  b) Neck

  c) Tubercle

- **Sternal Extremity**

  a) Slightly enlarged and roughened at the junction with the costal cartilage

- **The ribs** consist of both bony and cartilaginous sections.
- The more caudal ribs, known as "**false ribs**," form a costal arch by joining together, while the more cranial ribs, called "**true ribs**," connect directly to the sternum through costal cartilages at the costochondral junction.
- **Floating ribs**, in contrast, do not attach to either the costal arch or the sternum.
- The head of the rib is positioned more ventrally and typically articulates with one or two vertebral bodies. The surface where the articulation occurs is called the articular facet.
- The tubercle of the rib is located more dorsally and articulates with the transverse process of the thoracic vertebra.

Rib (Vertebral extremity)

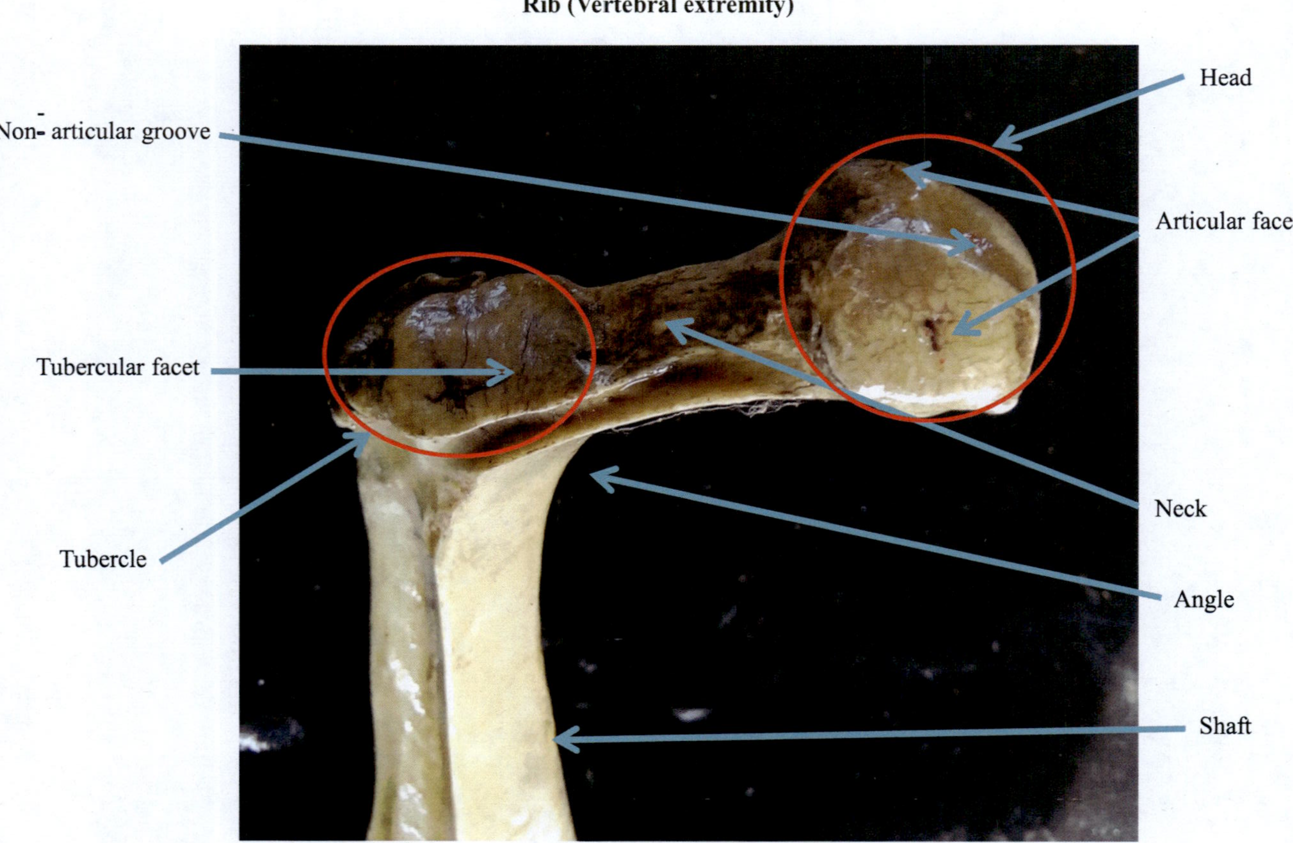

Ribs

- **Two Surfaces**

  a) Lateral (Convex)

  b) Medial (flattened from edge to edge)

- Borders

  a) Cranial (concave)

  b) Caudal (convex)

- The first rib is almost vertical
- **The mediastinum** is the central compartment of the thoracic cavity, located between the two pleural cavities.
- It contains several vital structures, including the thymus, thoracic lymph nodes, heart, aorta, trachea, esophagus, vagus nerves, and various other nerves and blood vessels.
- The mediastinum is divided into several regions: cranial, middle and caudal portion
- **Cranial part:** Contains the thymus.
- **Middle portion:** Houses the heart.
- **Dorsal and caudal parts:** Contain the esophagus, aorta, and caudal mediastinal lymph nodes.
- **Tracheobronchial lymph nodes:** Located at the junction of the trachea and bronchi, at the boundary of the mediastinal and pleural cavities.

Rib (Lateral surface)

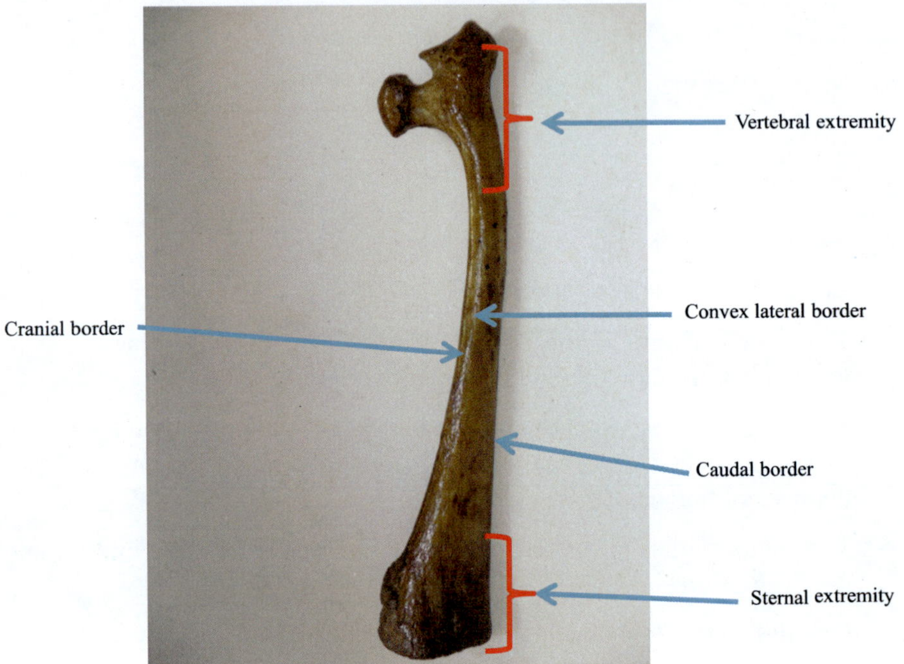

- **The caudal mediastinal lymph nodes** are located in the dorsal part of the caudal thoracic cavity, near the esophagus and aorta.
- These lymph nodes can become infected and enlarged, often as a result of pneumonia.
- If they swell significantly, they may compress nearby structures, such as the dorsal vagal trunk, which is responsible for innervating the rumen in cattle. This can lead to symptoms like bloat, "**vagal indigestion**," and weight loss.

Rib (Medial surface)

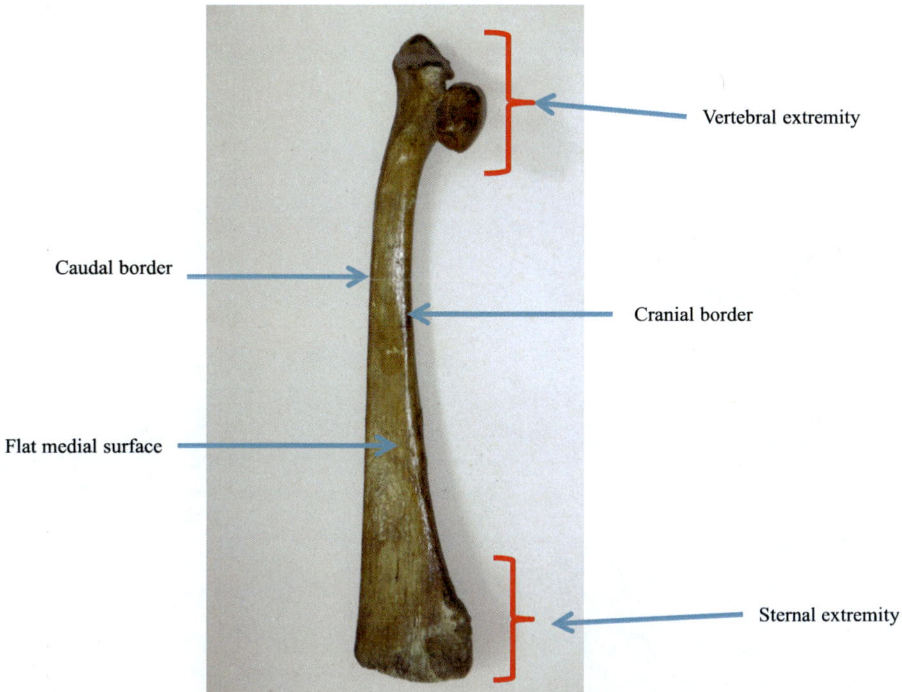

- Bovine animals have **fibrous and resilient connective tissue** in the pleura that forms the boundaries of the mediastinum.
- This anatomical feature helps prevent the spread of conditions from the mediastinum to the pleural cavities or between the two pleural cavities.
- It also facilitates standing thoracic and pericardial surgeries in cattle.
- Injuries to the axillary region can result in pneumomediastinum.
- In large animals, the **costal arch** (the edge of the rib cage) is positioned more caudally, while the lung field is located more cranially, particularly in ruminants.
- In bovines, the abdominal contents extend cranially into the thoracic cavity and are located beneath the caudal-most ribs.

Rib (Sternal extremity)

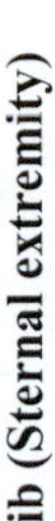

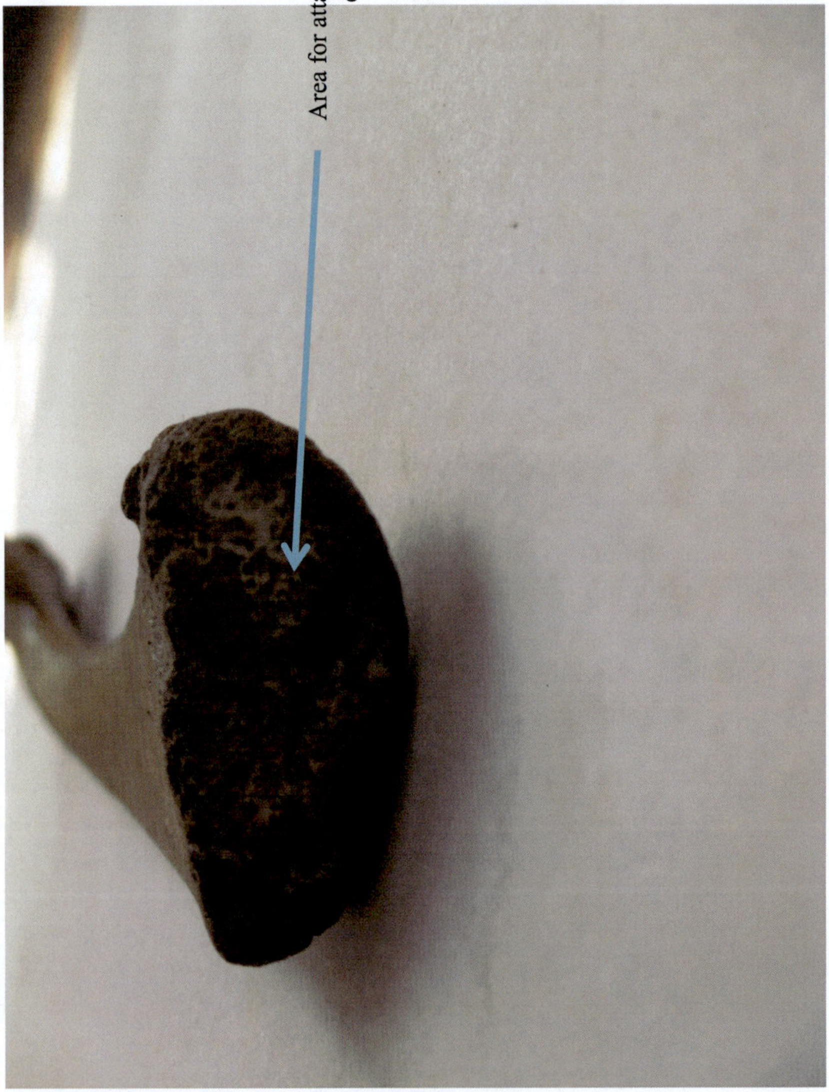

Area for attachment with costal cartilage

- When performing a physical exam, it's important to auscultate the lung fields cranially in cattle due to their **unique thoracic structure**.
- The heart fields and cardiac notches should also be noted on both the left and right sides of large animals.
- For **thoracentesis**, the needle or trocar must be inserted carefully to avoid lung tissue, often using ultrasound for guidance.
- In cattle, the **steeper pleural reflection**, due to their shorter and deeper thorax, must be considered when choosing the insertion site.
- **Auscultation** in cattle is a vital diagnostic technique used to evaluate the heart, lungs, and ruminal sounds. It involves listening to internal body sounds with a stethoscope to detect abnormalities, such as heart murmurs, lung sounds, or rumen.
- The area for auscultation and percussion of the heart in cattle is located between the 3rd and 5th intercostal spaces on the left side.
- For the lungs, the **auscultation and percussion** area forms a triangular shape, with the following boundaries: The caudal angle of the scapula cranially, the olecranon process of the ulna inferiorly, the 11th intercostal space caudally.

Sternum

- Seven Sternebre
- Two Surfaces (Dorsal and Ventral)
- Cranial extremity, the manubrium sterni or Presternum
- The body or mesosterni presents laterally at the junction of the segments, concave facets for articulation with the cartilages of the sternal ribs
- The Caudal extremity or metasternum presents the xiphoid cartilage

Sternum (Ventral Surface)

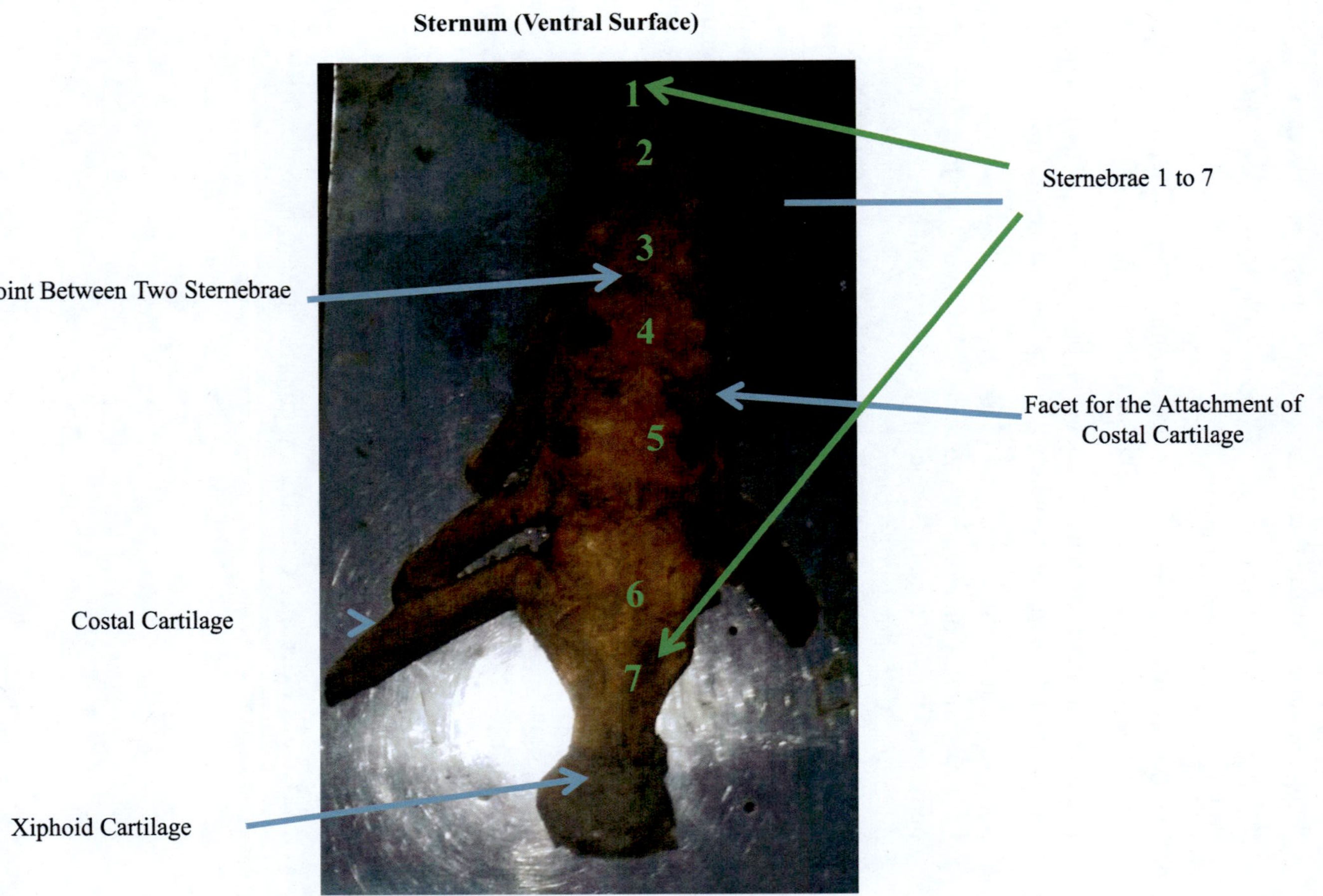

- In cattle, **the sternum** has eight articular cavities for connecting with the first eight costal cartilages.
- The first cavity is located on the cranial aspect of the first sternebra, with the remaining cavities between the sternebrae.
- **The manubrium** sterni (presternum) forms the cranial part of the sternum, while the **xiphoid cartilage** (metasternum) forms the caudal end.
- The diaphragm attaches to the xiphoid cartilage, which helps form the floor of the abdomen.
- The ventral surface of the xiphoid cartilage also provides attachment for the transverse abdominis and linea alba muscles.
- The body of the sternum, or mesosternum, lies between the manubrium and xiphoid cartilage.

Recumbent cow

- The term "recumbent cow" refers to a cow that is late in pregnancy or has recently calved, and is lying down (either on her chest or side) unable to stand.
- This condition is considered a veterinary emergency and requires immediate attention and intensive care.
- Nursing a recumbent cow can be physically demanding and time-consuming.
- Without prompt and proper care, the cow may suffer from secondary complications, regardless of the underlying cause of her inability to rise. Therefore, timely intervention is crucial to prevent further harm and ensure recovery.